PHYSIOLOGY - LABORATORY AND CLINICAL RESEARCH

BONE LOSS

RISK FACTORS, DETECTION AND PREVENTION

Physiology - Laboratory and Clinical Research

Additional books in this series can be found on Nova's website under the Series tab.

Additional e-books in this series can be found on Nova's website under the e-book tab.

Human Anatomy and Physiology

Additional books in this series can be found on Nova's website under the Series tab.

Additional e-books in this series can be found on Nova's website under the e-book tab.

PHYSIOLOGY - LABORATORY AND CLINICAL RESEARCH

BONE LOSS

RISK FACTORS, DETECTION AND PREVENTION

KUO-CHENG LU
EDITOR

New York

For permission to use material from this book please contact us:
Telephone 631-231-7269; Fax 631-231-8175
Web Site: http://www.novapublishers.com

Additional color graphics may be available in the e-book version of this book.

Library of Congress Cataloging-in-Publication Data

ISBN: 978-1-62417-169-7
Library of Congress Control Number: 2012950905

Published by Nova Science Publishers, Inc. † New York

CONTENTS

PREFACE

The past several decades have seen dramatic advances in understanding the pathogenesis of osteoporosis. The science of bone loss disease has progressed steadily from a discipline focused largely on metabolic bone physiology, through successive eras of cellular and molecular biology, and now into molecular mapping and personalized medicine. During that time, the processes which initiate and mediate bone loss have emerged with increasing clarity and complexity from early perceptions that they reflected largely increased osteoclast activity.

This book "Bone Loss: Risk Factors, Detection and Prevention" is produced not only to provide a comprehensive review of current understanding of the pathophysiology of bone loss, but also contribute a series of well selected individual updated chapters that provide snapshots of the bone science in specified population. The comprehensive book perfectly arranged into eight sections. An in depth review of systemic chronic kidney disease-related syndrome "Chronic kidney disease-mineral and bone disorder" (CKD-MBD) in chronic kidney disease and end-stage renal disease population is done by Kuo-Cheng Lu, et al in the first chapter. In the second session, Chang-Hsun Hsieh and Dee-Pei reviewed the risk factors, prevention and therapeutic approaches to bone loss in diabetes population. The factors influencing bone loss in cardiovascular disease population are extensively reviewed by Jen-Yu Wang and Kuo-Cheng Lu in section 3. The topic is followed by an interesting one which introduces the mechanisms of bone loss in prostate cancer by Carsten Goessl, et al. In chapter 5, the role of hormone, prolactin in bone loss is discussed by Erika C. O. Naliato. A new concept on inflammation, immune and microbial mechanism of bone resorption was extensively revised by Garlet GP et al. in chapter 6. A great discovery of bone protection by green tea is published in chapter 7 by Noboru Hasegawa et al. from Japan. Hip fracture, an important health and economic impact in elder population all over the world, was revised in detail by J.D. Pedrera-Zamorano et al. in the last chapter.

The reader of "Bone Loss: Risk Factors, Detection and Prevention" will find something of interest to all students and research investigators of bone loss disease in the form of assembled scientific reviews and updates that make up this book. As in all good stories, the best comes last when the material presented here is integrated into the clinical and treatment aspects of bone loss that are covered in the book "Bone Loss: Risk Factors, Detection and Prevention".

In: Bone Loss
Editor: Kuo-Cheng Lu
ISBN: 978-1-62417-169-7

Chapter 1

BONE LOSS IN CHRONIC KIDNEY DISEASE

***Kuo-Cheng Lu*[1], *Cai-Mei Zheng*[2], *Chia-Chao Wu*[3] *and Pauling Chu*[3]**

[1]Division of Nephrology, Department of Medicine,
Cardinal Tien Hospital, School of Medicine,
Fu Jen Catholic University,
New Taipei City, Taiwan
[2]Division of Nephrology, Department of Internal Medicine,
Shuang Ho Hospital, Taipei Medical University,
Taipei, Taiwan
[3]Division of Nephrology, Department of Medicine,
Tri-Service General Hospital, National Defense Medical Center,
Taipei, Taiwan

ABSTRACT

Patients with chronic kidney disease (CKD) often develop "chronic kidney disease-mineral and bone disorder" (CKD-MBD). This systemic CKD-related syndrome is manifested by complex abnormalities in bone and mineral metabolism—including bone lesions referred to as renal osteodystrophy (ROD)—and/or extraskeletal calcification. Disruptions in mineral metabolism and bone microarchitecture occur early in the course of CKD, typically beginning as a high bone turnover rate resulting from secondary hyperparathyroidism (SHPT). The condition worsens with the progressive decline in kidney function, as the high bone turnover leads to reduced bone mineral density (BMD) during the course of chronic renal failure. Patients with SHPT exhibit preferential loss of cortical bone (e.g., the distal radius and the femoral neck), often with preserved or slightly increased cancellous bone (e.g., the lumbar spine).

Several factors impact the progression of CKD-MBD. In CKD stages 3 and 4, patients with diabetes have lower cortical bone BMD when compared with non-diabetic patients. Calcium load also has a negative impact on the progression of vascular calcification in dialysis patients with adynamic bone disease. Low bone volume is associated with increased coronary calcifications in patients on dialysis, with the degree of risk dependent on the patient's age and dialysis duration. Regular treatments with heparin or anti-platelet drugs also impact BMD in hemodialysis (HD) patients. Low BMD is a major risk factor for hip fracture, and this risk is exacerbated in patients undergoing peritoneal dialysis (PD), who show a significant reduction in cortical BMD. Following kidney transplantation, the greatest rates of bone loss and increased fracture rates are observed in the first 6-18 months, caused by both pre-transplantation bone disease and immunosuppressive therapy.

Various medical treatments for SHPT can improve bone mass. Patients with refractory SHPT may require a parathyroidectomy (PTX), which provides marked, sustained improvements in BMD. Markers of bone turnover can predict how PTX will change BMD. Renal osteodystrophy can't be assessed by BMD measurements alone; the gold standard for ROD diagnosis is based on histomorphological changes revealed by bone biopsy. However, because of technical difficulties and a lack of testing facilities, it is often more convenient to use several serum bone markers to measure changes in bone turnover. The combined use of BMD and marker measurements may be a valuable approach in clinical practice.

1. Fracture Risk in Patients with CKD

1.1. Bone Turnover in CKD

Bone turnover occurs in both cortical and trabecular bone, with a relatively higher turnover rate in trabecular bone, representing the bone mineralization process. Stages of bone remodeling include osteoclast resorption, reversal, maturation of osteoblasts, osteoid or unmineralized bone formation, mineralization, and finally a quiescent stage. During normal bone mineralization, calcium phosphate crystals are produced by bone-forming cells and precise amounts are laid within the bone fibrous matrix. This important step is orchestrated by a tightly coupled group of osteoclasts and osteoblasts to continuously replace old bone with new bone.

The bone remodeling process occurs through the actions of osteoprotegerin (OPG) and the RANK (receptor activator of nuclear factor κB) system, which is regulated by hormones (PTH, calcitriol, estrogen, and glucocorticoids), cytokines, and interleukins. Circulating parathyroid hormones (PTH) increase the eroded surface, osteoid surface, and mineralizing surface — subsequently increasing the numbers of osteoclasts and osteoblasts. Calcitriol increases bone mineralization by stimulating intestinal calcium and phosphorus absorption; it also promotes osteoblast differentiation and stimulates osteoblast expression of cytokines, including bone-specific alkaline phosphatase, osteocalcin, osteonectin, OPG, etc. Dentin matrix protein 1, bone sialoprotein, phosphoprotein kinases, and alkaline phosphatase also play roles in the mineralization process [1].

Coordinated bone remodeling may be up or down regulated by systemic hormones (PTH, calcitriol) or local factors [interleukins (IL-1, IL-6) and growth factors (tumor necrosis factor-α, IGF)]. In high turnover (hyperparathyroid) renal osteodystrophy (ROD) , serum PTH increases the levels of receptor activator of nuclear factor kB ligand (RANKL), which are significantly higher in HD patients. A clinical study carried out by Avbersek-Luznik et al. demonstrated that PTH-enhanced bone resorption occurs via a mechanism involving increased RANKL synthesis [2]. RANK-RANKL interaction provides essential signals to osteoclast progenitors, leading to osteoclast differentiation, an important step in osteoclastogenesis, and bone resorption. This process can be blocked by osteoprotegerin (OPG), a decoy receptor for RANKL that protects against bone resorption and extensive deterioration. Increased PTH level is also associated with muscle dysfunction, immune disturbances, negative cardiac inotropic effects, higher fasting serum insulin and triglyceride levels, and impaired hematopoiesis [3-5]. Observational studies have found PTH levels of >400-600 pg/mL to be significantly associated with mortality [6, 7].

1.2. Bone Density, Fracture, and Mortality in CKD

Osteoporosis is the most prevalent condition leading to low-trauma fractures in humans worldwide. Many metabolic disturbances, including renal bone disorders, lead to osteoporosis and the pathologic fractures associated with osteoporosis, as well as non-osteoporotic fragility fractures. Osteoporosis can be part of the impaired bone quality (altered architecture, remodeling, mass, and volume) seen in CKD-MBD patients; however, despite this overlap, osteoporosis and CKD-MBD progress via distinct pathways, each resulting in impaired bone strength and higher risk of low-trauma fracture.

The prevalence of osteoporosis varies according to CKD stage. Early CKD patients, from stages 1 through 3, do not exhibit altered bone strength or pathological fractures according to any prospective or observational data, even with the presence of mildly elevated PTH level and intermittent hyperphosphatemia. Thus, any fracture in these early CKD stages is mostly associated with osteoporosis, rather than CKD-MBD. Derangements in phosphorus, PTH, or bone turnover markers, or bone histomorphometry associated with CKD-MBD can be seen as early at stage 3 CKD. Most patients with stage 4 and 5 CKD exhibit alternations in bone quality due to metabolic bone disorders and/or decreases in BMD [8, 9]; at the time of initiation of dialysis, up to 50% of patients have had a fracture [10, 11]. Furthermore, CKD patients are more commonly associated with poor nutrition, inactivity, myopathy, and peripheral neuropathy, which altogether play a role in muscle weakness and falls [12]. A study conducted by Huang et al. revealed that advanced age, low body weight, low serum albumin level, and high ALP and iPTH levels were associated with low bone mass in hemodialysis patients [13].

CKD is associated with higher morbidity and mortality fractures. The Third National Health and Nutrition Examination Survey of 6,270 men and women showed a two-fold increased risk of hip fracture in those with an estimated glomerular filtration rate (eGFR) < 60 mL/min, as compared to those with an eGFR ≥ 60 mL/min [14]. The Study of Osteoporotic Fractures surveyed 9,704 women of 65 years and older, and revealed a 1.5-fold increased hip fracture risk among those with an eGFR between 45-50 mL/min and a 2-fold increase among women with an eGFR < 45 mL/min, when compared to women with an eGFR ≥ 60 mL/min [15]. Another cross-sectional study conducted on 5,481 elderly men and women also revealed that those with an eGFR < 65 mL/min had an approximate 1.5-fold increased risk of hip, spine, and wrist fractures, compared to those with eGFR > 65 mL/min [16]. The incidence of fractures increases with advanced CKD stage and is highest in stage 5 CKD patients on dialysis. A large retrospective study based on data from the United States Renal Data System (USRDS) showed an increased relative risk of hip fracture in both men and women with stage 5 CKD on dialysis, compared to the general population [17]. After suffering a hip fracture, these stage 5 CKD patients on dialysis also had an increased 1-year mortality rate of 64%, as compared to the 15–20% 1-year mortality rate in the general population; this patient group also tended to experience hip fracture at a younger age compared with the general population (16 and 13 years earlier among men and women, respectively) [18]. Knowing which patients are at a higher risk for fractures and falls among CKD patients may enable the establishment of protocols to decrease the economic costs, morbidity, and mortality associated with fractures in this patient group. In CKD patients with severe pathological fractures, assessment of bone markers and, in some cases, bone biopsy may be needed to diagnose CKD-MBD with osteoporosis, which may influence the prescribed pharmacological therapies.

1.3. Relationship between BMD and Renal Osteodystrophy

Renal osteodystrophy (ROD) includes a variety of bone lesions that differ in both mechanisms of development and therapeutic approaches. The TMV (turnover, mineralization, and volume) system is a recently developed, simple, and clinically comprehensive system to classify CKD-MBD [19]. The TMV system provides information on the range of pathologic abnormalities that can occur in CKD patients. Bone turnover and bone volume can be classified as high, normal, or low. Bone mineralization is classified as normal or abnormal. The Kidney Disease Outcomes Quality Initiative (K/DOQI) guidelines distinguish the following six types of bone disorders on the basis of TMV system: hyperparathyroid bone disease (high turnover, normal mineralization, and any bone volume), mixed bone disease (high turnover with mineralization defect and normal bone volume), osteomalacia (low-turnover bone with abnormal mineralization and low-to-medium bone volume), adynamic bone disease (low-turnover bone with normal mineralization and low or normal bone volume), amyloid bone disease, and aluminum bone disease [20-22].

The types of bone histology depend on the degree and duration of renal impairment, patient age and comorbidities, mode and years of dialysis, associated medications for hyperparathyroidism, serum calcium and phosphate levels, etc. In addition to ROD, these patients are also more likely than the general population to have osteoporosis, which is also influenced by age, gender, menopausal status, drugs, nutrition, and exercise [23]. Thus, it is difficult to separate these disease entities clinically.

The most common high turnover abnormality in ROD is hyperparathyroid bone disorder (HPBD; osteitis fibrosa cystica: OFC) with excessive osteoclastic bone resorption and bone marrow fibrosis [24]. HPBD (Figure 1) may present with several types of radiographic findings. Due to increased osteoclastic activity, bone resorption may occur in many skeletal sites, including subperiosteal, intracortical, endosteal, trabecular, subchondral, and subligamentous, etc [25]. Subperiosteal bone resorption is most commonly occur in the phalanges, humerus, and distal epiphyseal region of clavicles [26]. Subchondral resorption in sacroiliac joints may lead to “pseudo-widening” of the joint. Losses of lamina dura of the teeth are also common in SHPT patients [25]. Excessive osteoblastic activity may follows as compensation for the bone resorption, with resultant osteosclerosis [25], which is commonly seen in most sites of axial skeleton, including the pelvis, ribs, spine, and skull. Excessive osteoid accumulation below the endplates of vertebral bodies occurs and with normal density in the middle parts, these vertebral bodies appear under radiological films as “rugger jersey spine sign” [27]. Excessive terminal phalanges resorption may result in a deformity known as acroosteolysis [25]. Brown tumors, known to be caused by rapid osteoclastic activity and peritrabecular fibrosis, may affect pelvis, ribs, clavicles and sometimes may result in pathological fractures. Brown tumors of vertebral column may also present with spinal cord compression [28, 29]. Metastatic calcification, a result of increased calcium/phosphate solubility product in extracellular fluid [30], is responsible for the vascular calcification in SHPT patients. Metastatic calcifications mostly affect the hips and shoulders, although other joints may also be affected [31, 32].

Low-turnover bone diseases include osteomalacia, aluminum-induced bone disease, and adynamic bone disease (ABD) (Figure 2). Osteomalacia alone is an uncommon presentation in HD patients [33]. This mineralization defect is related to reduced 1,25-dihydroxyvitamin D and chronic metabolic acidosis [34]. Aluminum ingestion causes a mineralization defect, markedly reduces both osteoclast resorption and osteoblast surface, and is associated with the low-bone turnover disease osteomalacia. Chronic low-dose aluminum exposure with high intake of vitamin D in dialysis patients reduces parathyroid hormone synthesis and secretion, even in the presence of hyperphosphatemia; these patients may present with adynamic bone disease rather than osteomalacia[35]. The prevalence of aluminum-related bone disorders has been reduced over recent decades due to emergence of non-aluminum-containing dialysate solutions and phosphate binders [36].

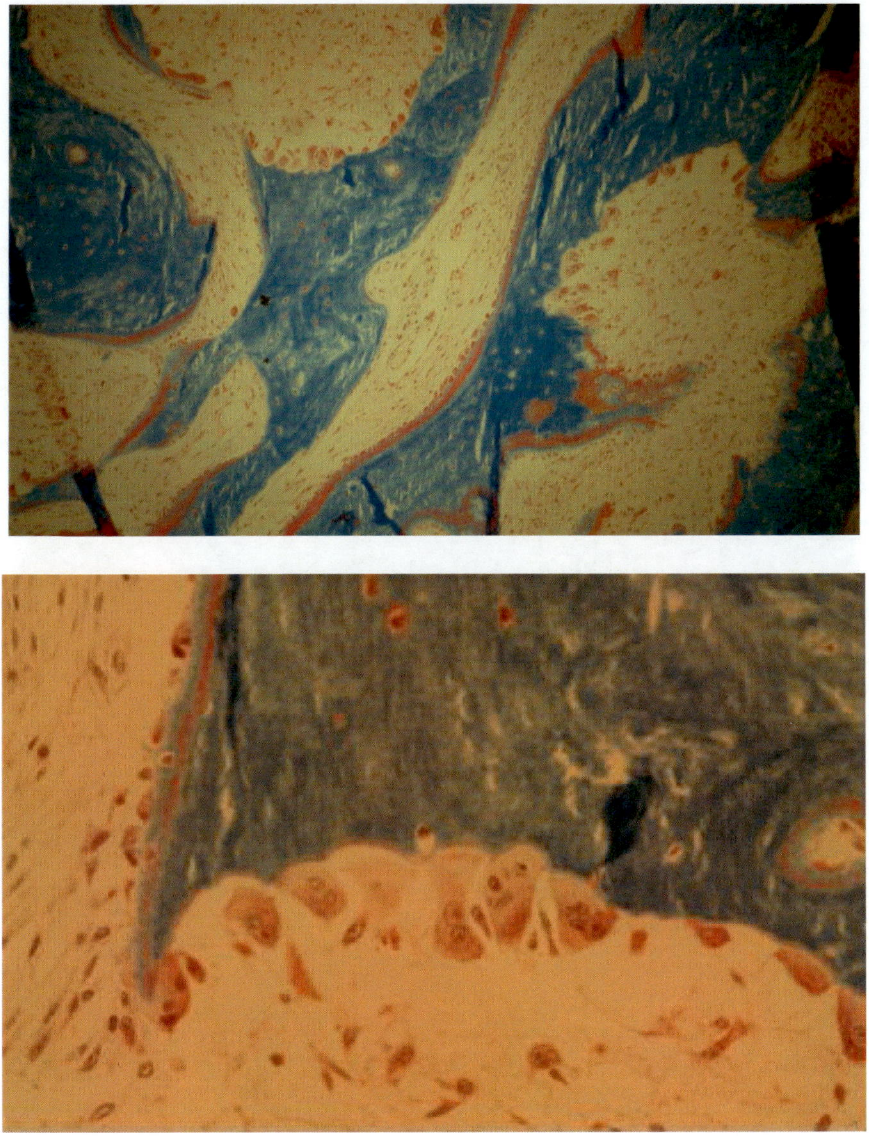

Figure 1. Histology of bone showing hyperparathyroid bone disorders (HPBD). (Fibrosis and prominent osteoclast resorption are seen).

2. CKD Progression and BMD Changes

2.1. Low BMD in CKD not yet Receiving Dialysis

With progressive decline in renal function, CKD patients suffer from hyperparathyroidism secondary to a decrease in serum calcium, a reduction in 1,25-$(OH)_2$-vitamin D (calcitriol) synthesis, and/or impaired phosphate excretion. The cloning of klotho and fibroblast growth factor 23 (FGF-23) has enabled the progressive unraveling of their roles in calcium/phosphate metabolism over the past decade. Progressive P accumulation leads to increases in serum PTH and FGF-23, both of which play important roles in consequences like renal osteodystrophy, hyperparathyroidism, calcemic uremic arteriopathy, and uremic cardiomyopathy.

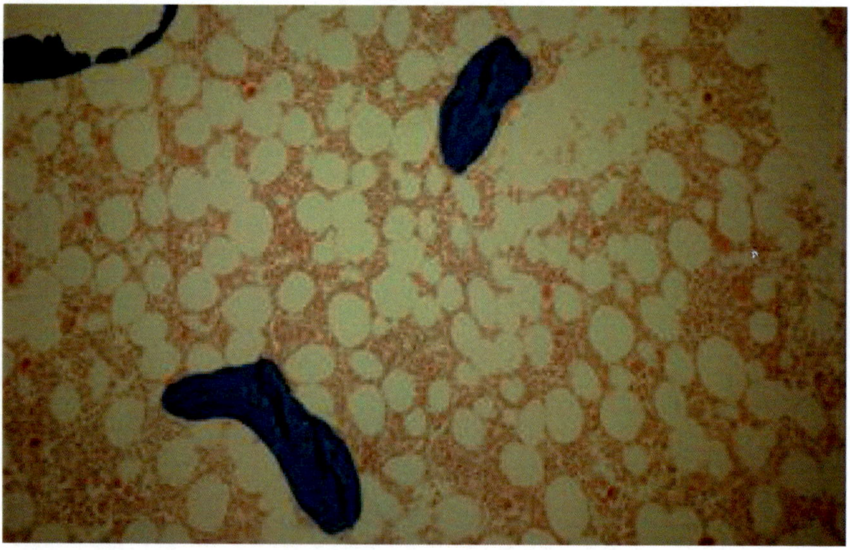

Figure 2. Histology of bone showing adynamic disorders (ABD). (Decreased bone turnover rate: lack of osteoblast activity and defective osteoid mineralization).

Normal serum phosphorus and calcium levels are maintained by the integrative actions of parathyroid hormone (PTH) and 1,25-dihydroxyvitamin D3 (calcitriol). The phosphatonin fibroblast growth factor-23 (FGF-23) directly controls renal phosphorus excretion and, along with the aforementioned hormones, plays a role in regulating systemic mineral metabolism. FGF-23, a 25-amino acid protein, prevents renal phosphate reclamation by decreasing the type 2a sodium-dependent phosphate co-transporters (NaPi-2a) expression in PCT. FGF-23 also suppresses the expression of 1α-hydroxylase, the enzyme that converts 25-hydroxyvitamin D3 to calcitriol, resulting in decreased renal production of activated vitamin D [37-39]. FGF 23 and FGF receptor interaction is facilitated by the co-receptor Klotho [40]. Serum FGF-23 levels are found to be increased as early as CKD stage 3, which helps to keep serum P within the normal laboratory range. FGF-23 may also be responsible for early reduction in calcitriol levels during early CKD [41-43]. These findings indicate that clinical strategies to decrease FGF-23 may be therapeutically useful for normalizing calcitriol levels in these patients. Hasegawa et al. [44] found significantly increased FGF23 levels in CKD rats as compared with the normal rats, as early as 10 days after kidney destruction, preceding the rises of phosphate and creatinine. The factors that lead to this early FGF23 elevation are unknown.

Further loss of renal tissue leads to reduced Klotho expression, resulting in FGF resistance and correspondingly increased serum FGF level. This frequently occurs in stage 4 and 5 CKD, when hyperphosphatemia persists despite marked elevations of FGF-23 and PTH [45]. Hyperphosphatemia eventually becomes clinically significant due to many factors, including diminished nephron mass [46], FGF-23 resistance, and reduced calcitriol synthesis. The accumulated P combined with Ca results in calcium phosphate crystal deposition in soft tissue. Hypocalcemia, hyperphosphatemia, and low calcitriol levels all stimulate PTH formation and secretion, known as secondary hyperparathyroidism [47]. Excessive skeletal remodeling occurs in secondary hyperparathyroidism during progressive CKD, resulting in excessive bone resorption, defective bone formation, and abnormal mineralization. Finally, defective bone mineralization with heterotopic mineralization or metastatic calcification occurs in blood vessels and heart tissue, also known as calcific uremic arteriolopathy (CUA) [48, 49].

Patients with CKD have reduced BMD due to multifactorial causes, including acid-base disturbances, and impaired vitamin D and parathyroid hormone (PTH) homeostasis. Chronic metabolic acidosis in CKD patients may increase bone resorption due to bone buffering and slow dissolution of bone mineral [50]. Bone biopsies of mild to moderate CKD patients reveal PTH excess and increased bone turnover [51]. Bone turnover markers have been found to correlate with PTH levels and GFR [52], and low calcitriol level is found to be a independent risk factor for hip fractures [15]. Although many studies reported a decrease BMD in CKD patients, the exact relationship between BMD and CKD was still unclear due to study limitations [53]. In the Third National Health and Nutrition Examination Survey (NHAHES-III) Study, subjects with worse renal function had significantly lower femoral BMD; however, this association was explained by confounding factors, like age, sex, ethnicity, etc. Renal function itself was not found to be independently associated with BMD after taking sex, age, and body weight into account [54].

2.2. Influence of Comorbidities

CKD is a complex comorbid condition with a multiplicity of clinical manifestations. It is closely linked with cardiovascular disease and associated with a very high mortality rate. In the United States, CKD consumes about one-third of Medicare expenditures. Co-morbid conditions of CKD include hypertension, diabetes, dyslipidemia, cardiovascular disease, anemia, and bone and mineral disorders. Changes in mineral metabolism with alterations of hormonal regulation have recently been found in CKD, associated with various forms of bone diseases; this has become known as the kidney-bone axis. During the past decade, investigators have focused more on the bone-vascular axis, and the relationship between mineral metabolism disorders and soft tissue and cardiovascular calcifications.

The complex pathophysiologic mechanisms of arterial calcification include disturbances of mineral metabolism and mineral-regulating proteins. Longitudinal population-based studies reveal an association between progressive vascular calcifications (VC) and bone demineralization. In dialysis patients, coronary artery calcification score was found to be inversely correlated with vertebral bone mass. In other words, increasing arterial stiffness co-exists with progressive bone loss, which is responsible for most of the cardiovascular events in CKD patients. Vascular calcification is an active process involving various proteins that are similar to those involved in bone and mineral metabolism [55, 56]; this process represents a part of CKD-mineral and bone disorder [19].

Risk factors for premature VC in end-stage renal disease (ESRD) patients differ from the traditional atherogenic risk factors. Hyperparathyroidism and alterations in Ca-P mineral metabolism, especially hyperphosphatemia, modulate both renal osteodystrophy and vascular calcification [57, 58]. An association has been observed between extraosseous calcifications and hyperparathyroidism [59, 60] and reversal of extraosseous calcifications with reduction of bone turnover after parathyroidectomy [61-63]. In contrast, one study described an association between low bone turnover and vascular calcifications [64]. Therapeutic measures for SHPT—like PTX and excessive calcium or aluminum load, which lead to lower bone turnover and adynamic bone disease—may also influence the development of arterial calcification [64]. A recent study carried out by Asci et al. [65] on 207 CKD stage 5 regular HD patients revealed an association between bone turnover, bone volume, and coronary calcifications. After adjusting for traditional risk factors (e.g., age, gender, DM, smoking, serum lipid, history of CVD, and hs-CRP) they found that low bone turnover was negatively correlated with coronary artery calcification (CAC), high bone turnover was positively correlated with CAC, and no association was found between normal turnover and CAC [65]. Age is a known risk factor for cardiovascular calcification in both general populations [67] and HD patients, and an interaction between cancellous bone volume and age was also found to be associated with CAC [66]. Thus, in addition to the demonstrated nonmodifiable risk factors (age, sex, diabetes mellitus, and HD duration), bone turnover and bone volume should also be considered as non-traditional risk factors that may influence CAC.

Diabetic ESRD patients tend to present with adynamic bone disease with or without aluminum deposition [68, 69], whereas present with hyperparathyroid bone disease in less than 10 percent of cases [70]. Bone resorption markers like serum tartrate-resistant acid phosphatase (TRAP) and urinary hydroxyproline are increased, especially when associated nephropathy develops. Insulin plays a role in bone anabolism through the insulin-like growth factor 1 (IGF-1) pathway. Patients with type 1 diabetes mellitus (DM) with true insulin deficiency may exhibit more bone loss than type 2 DM patients, in whom serum insulin levels are increased due to tissue resistance. Although bone mass can remain high in type 2 DM patients, bone quality is impaired due to accumulation of advanced glycation end products (AGE) in collagen. Increased bone fragility may also result from low bone turnover, reduced unmineralized bone matrix, and increased collagen glycosylation [71, 72]. Thus, bone density in these patients may not predict increased bone fragility [73]. Furthermore, diabetic ESRD patients often have other risk factors for fractures, including longer diabetes duration, diabetic retinopathy, neuropathy, and insulin treatment [74-77]. The regular oral hypoglycemic medications may also play a role in bone loss in these patients.

Metabolic syndrome (MS) is also associated with low bone mineral density (BMD) in patients with chronic kidney disease. Studies have shown that in both MS group and non-MS groups, BMD was negatively correlated with age, hemodialysis period, and parathormone (PTH) [78, 79].

2.3. Influence of Treatments (Medications) on CKD-related Osteodystrophy

Drug-induced osteoporosis is an important consideration in CKD patients. Unfractionated heparin (UFH) is the most common anticoagulant used in hemodialysis units, due to its relative ease of use, safety, and low cost; however, it is associated with many known side effects, such as heparin-induced thrombocytopenia, hypertriglyceridemia, and hyperkalemia. It is unclear whether intermittent heparin use is related to low bone mineral density, since most dialysis patients have other associated risk factors for osteoporosis, like diabetes mellitus, secondary hyperparathyroidism, old age, and physical inactivity. Therefore, UFH is only replaced with other anticoagulants (e.g., direct thrombin inhibitors, citrate dialysate, heparin-free dialysis) when other complications develop, such as heparin-induced thrombocytopenia. A study conducted by Grzegorzewska et al. [80] revealed that dialysis patients who receive regular LMWH, antiplatelet agents, or both, show lower bone mineral density in the femoral neck, but results of larger clinical trials are pending.

In diabetic CKD patients, skeletal effects of pharmacological treatments of type 2 diabetes also play a role in determining BMD. Biguanides like metformin increase the differentiation of bone marrow mesenchymal stem cells (MSC) into osteoblasts through the transactivation of Runt-related transcription factor 2 (RUNX2), resulting in increased bone formation. Glitazones, by simultaneously activating peroxisome proliferator-activating receptor γ (PPARγ) and inhibiting RUNX2, shift MSCs toward the adipocyte lineage, resulting in a reduced osteoblastic lineage [81].

Glucocorticoids are the drugs that most often cause osteoporotic fractures in both general and ESRD populations. Other medications have also been proven to be associated with bone loss, including calcineurin inhibitors, antiretroviral drugs, selective inhibitors of serotonin reuptake, anticonvulsants, loop diuretics, oral anticoagulants, and proton pump inhibitors. Cyclical hormone replacement therapy (HRT) may maintain BMD in postmenopausal women with secondary amenorrhea after dialysis [82]. Therapeutic measures like continuous hormone-replacement therapy (HRT), bisphosphonates, and selective estrogen receptor modulators (SERMS) may improve BMD in normal renal function status, but their roles in ESRD patients are still unclear.

2.4. Influence of Age and Gender

As the average age of CKD and ESRD patients increases, age-associated osteoporosis is also increased in these patients, at a higher rate than in general population. Age is an independent factor associated with bone loss in CKD and ESRD patients. Protein malnutrition, inflammation, and glucose abnormalities are more frequent in older ESRD populations, and are responsible for more BMD loss in this group compared with in younger patients. Postmenopausal osteoporosis is also a complication related to renal mineral and bone disorder. In a study including 112 postmenopausal hemodialysis patients, serum estradiol levels were found to be higher in hemodialysis patients than in those without CKD, and endogenous estrogen was found to play a role in preventing bone loss in postmenopausal hemodialysis women [83]. Many studies have found a high prevalence of calcidiol deficiency and insufficiency in predialysis patients, regardless of geographic location. A significant inverse correlation between calcidiol and parathyroid levels has also been noted in both general and predialysis populations, but the underlying mechanism underlying calcidiol deficiency is unknown [84].

Decreased physical activity may be associated with loss of bone strength in dialysis populations, and a rehabilitation program may play an important role in preventing this problem. Not only have high impact activities been proven osteogenic [85], but low-impact activities, like moderate intensity walking may also increase lumbar BMD [86]. Since CKD and ESRD patients are prone to fatigue and generally have a lower exercise capacity, low-impact activities are more favored in this population. A recent study revealed that active ESRD patients with adynamic bone disease have greater mineralized bone volume than less active patients [87]. Human studies including hemodialysis patients show a correlation between muscle strength and BMD [88]. The mechanical load applied by the muscle on bone is directly responsible for bone formation and remodeling [89]; therefore, simple, low-impact, weight-bearing exercises, such as walking and resistance exercise (strength training), are encouraged as daily physical activities in CKD patients to improve BMD.

3. Dialysis Modalities on BMD

BMD in Hemodialysis Patients

Even before dialysis, CKD patients with lower GFR (with or without higher iPTH values) present with lower BMD [90]. Prospective studies have revealed both gain and loss of BMD after the initiation of dialysis [91, 92], with increased dialysis associated with increased fracture risk. In HD patients, factors influencing low BMD include age, gender, lower body weight, and higher level of parathyroid hormone [93]. Compared to a general population, a dialysis patient population showed a 4.4-fold greater relative risk for hip fracture and a 2.4-fold higher mortality rate [18]. Risk factors like female gender, lower BMI, and white race influence hip joint fractures in the general population; however, in dialysis patients, lower serum iPTH values may indicate a greater risk of hip fractures [18]. Dialytic male patients seem to have higher risk of vertebral fractures, which is predicted by both BMD (a doubling prevalence for each 1-SD reduction in lumbar spine BMD) and by iPTH values [94]. Lower serum iPTH values are also associated with higher vertebral fracture prevalence; the serum iPTH values that predict the lowest fracture prevalence seem to be approximately one to three times the upper normal range [94].

Overall, osteoporosis is prevalent in hemodialysis patients. A cross-sectional study of hemodialysis patients using bone biopsy and histomorphometric analysis showed that hemodialytic osteoporosis patients have a low bone formation rate with normal bone eroded surface (BFR/BS), even with normal bone resorption. The results of this study are also alarming due to the fact that osteoporosis, a common disorder of aging, was determined to be prevalent in younger dialysis patients [95]. Cytokines that play roles in bone remodeling, like OPG, soluble receptor-activator of NF-κB ligand (sRANKL), and TNF-α, are also involved in the mechanisms of osteoporosis, in addition to many other traditional risk factors [95].

3.2. BMD in Peritoneal Dialysis Patients

The nature of bone disease differs in peritoneal dialysis (PD) patients and HD patients, since different factors influence calcium, phosphate, and PTH metabolism between the two modules. PD patients have better phosphorus clearance, higher removal of transferrin-bound aluminum, higher intake of phosphorus due to the recommended high protein diet, and higher bicarbonate loss than HD patients; they are also used to experiencing a constant glucose load and constant calcium load with regular or high calcium solutions [96]. PD patients are also more frequently associated with adynamic bone lesions (61% in PD patients vs. 36% in HD patients) [97, 98]. In PD patients, low BMD indicates poor outcome, since predictors of low BMD (age, poor nutrition status, metabolic acidosis, high phosphorus, anemia, etc.) are associated with worse prognosis in PD patients [99]. Low body weight seems to be the most important risk factor for osteoporosis in chronic PD patients [100]. Insufficient dialysis dose and older age also play an important role in osteoporosis of those patients. A recent cross-sectional study conducted by Jeong et al. evaluated the risk factors associated with BMD in chronic PD patients. Traditional markers of bone turnover (e.g., iPTH, 25-hydroxy (OH) vitamin D3, osteocalcin, bone alkaline phosphatase, and serum C-telopeptide) were not associated with BMD in PD patients, whereas nutritional markers (e.g., prealbumin, nPNA, and BMI) predicted BMD in chronic PD patients [101].

4. Renal Osteodystrophy

4.1. BMD in Secondary Hyperparathyroidism (SHPT)

4.1.1. Impact of SHPT on BMD

Increases in bone marrow fibrosis and both osteoblastic and osteoclastic activity occur in progressive SHPT. With increased bone resorption and defective mineralization, the resultant cortical bone thinning may lead to bone pain and/or pathological fractures. These types of high turnover bone lesions, including osteitis fibrosa and mixed uremic osteodystrophy, are common in patients with serum intact PTH levels over 400 pg/mL. The resultant increased bone remodeling may lead to reduced bone mineral density. The radius bone considered to be the site that correlates best with serum PTH levels in long-term dialyzed patients. In a prospective study of vitamin D deficiency and SHPT, high serum PTH was a significant predictor of mortality [102].

4.1.2. Medical Treatment of SHPT on BMD Change

Secondary hyperparathyroidism (SHPT) is responsible for many CKD-related consequences, such as renal osteodystrophy, extraskeletal calcification, and cardiovascular diseases. Treatments with vitamin D analogs, calcimimetics, and similar compounds; dietary phosphate restriction; and dialysis are important measures to prevent SHPT. Bisphosphonates, the usual osteoporotic medications, are not very effective in the setting of SHPT. The administration of calcium-containing phosphate binders and active vitamin D sterols is associated with development of hypercalcemia, hyperphosphatemia, adynamic osteodystrophy, and most importantly, with vascular calcifications. Hence, these older medications have been replaced with new calcium-free phosphate binders (e.g., sevelamer and lanthanum carbonate) that are used in combination with new active vitamin D sterols (e.g., doxercalciferol) for SHPT treatment. A prospective, randomized study demonstrated that sevelamer, when taken together with vitamin D analogs, may control PTH-induced bone disease as effectively as calcium carbonate, without increasing serum calcium concentration [103].

Supplementation with active vitamin D analogs was initially used to correct calcium/phosphorus disturbances in SHPT patients. Later, vitamin D treatment was also found to reduce cardiovascular mortality risk in dialysis patients, irrespective of intact-parathyroid hormone (iPTH) levels. In one of our studies, we revealed that calcitriol treatment in SHPT patients may attenuate inflammatory response, oxidative stress, and CD4+ T lymphocytes cytokines [104].

4.1.3. Surgical Treatment of SHPT on BMD Change

When SHPT is resistant to medical treatment, surgery may be required. Parathyroidectomy (PTX) is effective for long intervals as symptomatic therapy in cases of refractory SHPT that appear in uremic patients upon hemodialysis or after renal transplantation. In one study, we found serial biochemical marker changes to be associated with bone mineral density after PTX. The rapid decrease in iPTH levels after PTX was found to be related to suppression of bone resorption and improvement of bone formation. Baseline iPTH was positively correlated with BMD changes in femoral neck (FN) and lumbar spine (LS), as well as incremental changes in serum osteoprotegerin (OPG) levels [105]. Additionally, the increased serum OPG was positively related to the incremental changes in LS BMD, suggesting that inhibition of osteoclastic bone resorption may play an important role in improving BMD within the first year after PTX.

Studies in the investigation of serial changes in bone markers revealed that a rapid decrease in serum iPTH levels after PTX was related to suppression of bone resorption and improvement of bone formation. A transient, marked increase in serum alkaline phosphatase (Alk-P) was noted, peaking the second week after PTX. The baseline serum BAP, TRAP level, and femoral neck (FN) T-score predicted the amount of FN BMD improvement observed at 1 year after PTX. Furthermore, the baseline TRAP level and percent change in BAP at 2 weeks after PTX predicted changes in the LS T-score. These results indicated that the use of specific biochemical markers may benefit physicians and patients by providing reliable assessments of the success of surgery, and predictions of long-term changes in BMD after PTX [102] (Figure 3).

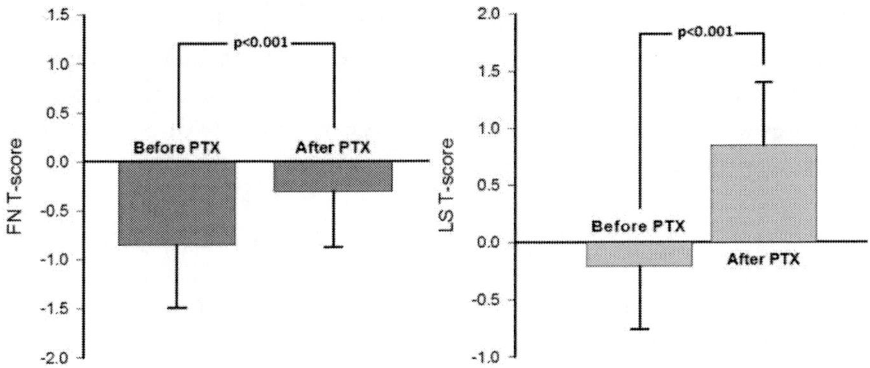

Figure 3. Parathyroidectomy improved bone mineralization in hemodialysis patients. Lumbar spine (LS) and femoral neck (FN) T-scores measured before and one year after parathyroidectomy (PTX). The plots show negative and positive T-scores, where Y=0 indicates the average level in a healthy 30-year old individual.[102]

4.2. BMD in Adynamic Bone Disorders (ABD)

Adynamic bone disease is a low-turnover bone lesion involving decreased osteoblast number and activity, with subsequent reduction in bone formation and activation frequency, as represented by an absence of osteoid accumulation in bone biopsies [106, 107]. The rate of collagen synthesis and the subsequent bone mineralization are subnormal, but mineralization defects are not prominent, with little marrow fibrosis. This finding distinguishes ABD from the other low-turnover bone form—osteomalacia—in which the mineralization defect exceeds the bone formation defect, and excessive osteoid is found [35] ABD is associated with suppression of PTH by exposure to calcium (generally as phosphate binders and dialysate fluid) and calcitriol. This type of ROD is more common in the elderly [108] and patients on chronic peritoneal dialysis. It is also associated with diabetes mellitus patients, in whom hyperglycemia and hypoinsulinemia act synergistically to inhibit PTH release [109]. ABD is associated with increased risk of developing vascular calcification, fractures [110] and calciphylaxis [111]. Dialysis patients with iPTH levels within the normal range have a 2-fold higher mortality risk than those with iPTH values ≥ three times the normal upper range. In these patients, lower iPTH values may reflect poor nutritional status [112], and may be associated with ABD and vascular calcification. Adynamic bone disease has become increasingly frequent since it has become possible to suppress PTH with calcium and potent vitamin D analogs. It has become increasingly common in dialysis centers with use of these medications, although the degree to which it increases morbidity and mortality is unknown. Intermittent bolus PTH infusions and other osteoporotic medicaitons, may be of possible benefit to patients with adynamic bone disease.

4.2.1. Effects of Medical Treatment for ABD on BMD Changes

Excessive use of calcium salts and calcitriol analogs should be avoided in ABD. Adynamic bone is treated by increasing bone turnover through an increase in PTH. This can best be accomplished by lowering doses of calcium-based phosphate binders and vitamin D, or entirely eliminating such therapy. The lowering of dialysate calcium (1.0 to 2.0 mEq/L) has also been suggested as a possible approach. The published study of this therapy in peritoneal dialysis patients led to a substantial increase in the number of patients with marked PTH elevation; however, this approach is still considered experimental [113, 114].

5. Kidney Transplantation

5.1. Effects of Pre-Transplantation Bone Disease

Successful renal transplantation may partially normalize bone and mineral metabolism. However, osteopenia and osteonecrosis are still important causes of long-term morbidity in transplant patients due to underlying renal osteodystrophy, diabetic bone disease, hypophosphatemia, and immunosuppression. Osteoporosis/osteopenia occurs more frequently during the first year post-transplantation (RTX). A study conducted among 70 Turkish patients after renal transplantation revealed that low BMI values and decreased vitamin D levels are independent risk factors for loss of bone mineral density in those patients [115]. Post-transplant bone disease is associated with both high and low serum iPTH levels. Hypophosphatemia occurring during the post-transplant period may lead to muscle weakness and occasionally osteomalacia. Painful leg syndrome and avascular bone necrosis are also observed during post-transplantation period.

Bone biopsy is necessary in the event of a disabling clinical outcome after transplantation, especially in patients who present with heterogeneous bone illness. Post-transplant bone loss mostly occurs in trabecular bone, although cortical bone may also be affected. A cross-sectional study using bone biopsy revealed that histopathological features of post-transplant osteopenia included osteoporosis-osteopenia, osteitis fibrosa, and osteomalacic lesions [116].

Since CKD patients are mostly associated with renal osteodystrophy, and substantial bone loss occurs during the first month of the post-operative period, it is important to predict bone mass and fracture risk at the time of renal transplantation. In uremia patients, HD duration and iPTH level must be considered in addition to other predictors of osteoporosis. Since post-transplant persistent hyperparathyroidism and hypercalcemia, and subsequent vascular calcifications may result from pre-transplant severe SHPT, it is crucial to control SHPT during the pre-transplant period.

5.2. Effects of Immunosuppressants

Glucocorticoid-induced osteoblast suppression and increased osteoclast activity lead to bone resorption in both the early and late post-transplant periods. Other glucocorticoid effects include decreased calcium absorption, suppression of gonadal hormone production [117], decreased insulin-like growth factor-1 (IGF-1) production, decreased sensitivity to PTH, increased receptor activator of NF-κB ligand (RANKL), and promotion of mesenchymal stem cell differentiation toward adipocytes instead of osteoblasts [118]. Steroid dosage is negatively related to low bone volume and turnover.

Increased bone turnover is also seen with the calcineurin inhibitors cyclosporine and tacrolimus; however, studies show no difference in bone loss among cyclosporine and tacrolimus users. In addition to osteopenia and osteonecrosis, increased plasma cyclosporine levels are related to possible intraosseous vasoconstriction and bone pain.

Since glucocorticoid exposure is the main factor contributing to bone loss after transplantation [119], newer immunosuppressive protocols with steroid-free regimens, more rapid steroid tapering, or lower steroid maintenance dosage represent important strategies to preserve BMD in transplant patients.

6. Serum Bone Turnover Markers

Although bone biopsy remains the gold standard for differentiating different forms of renal osteodystrophy, it is often reluctant for many physicians due to invasive, painful and often refused by many patients. Many noninvasive methods including biological bone markers are studied to assess bone metabolism. In chronic renal failure patients, several serum markers of metabolism are known, bone-specific alkaline phosphatase (bAP), procollagen type I carboxy-terminal extension peptide (PICP), procollagen type I cross-linked carboxy-terminal telopeptide (ICTP), pyridinoline(PYD), osteocalcin, and tartrate-resistant acid phosphatase (TRAP), etc.

6.1. Bone Resorption Markers

In end-stage renal disease (ESRD) and chronic hemodialysis patients, serum iPTH levels between 150 and 300 pg/mL are considered adequate. Four- to eight-fold elevations of PTH may predict high-turnover bone disease and be present in cases of HPBD. Bone loss in ROD patients may be predicted by the elevation of bone turnover markers. Elevation of serum TRACP-5b and total i-PTH strongly predicts radial cortical bone loss in dialysis patients [121]. However, since most CKD patients reveal relative resistance to PTH, and have other factors influencing PTH-bone axis (e.g., hyperphosphatemia, diabetes, age, gender, and use of vitamin D analogs), the validity of serum parathyroid hormone (i-PTH) as a surrogate marker is limited. Since a significant correlation between level of TRAP 5b and iPTH exists, TRAP 5b was now regarded as an important marker of bone resorption rate in ROD patients clinically. Urinary collagen N-terminal telopeptide X (NTX), a bone collagen degradation product, is positively correlated with iPTH and BSAP, and is regarded as a promising bone resorption marker in CKD patients. Furthermore, urine NTX also measures bone loss secondary to osteoporosis [122].

Sclerostin, a soluble inhibitor of osteoblast function, is associated with decreased bone turnover in dialysis patients, and one study revealed high sclerostin levels in dialysis patients with higher bone density. It remains to be determined whether its increase in dialysis patients has direct pathogenetic relevance or is only a secondary phenomenon remains [123].

6.2. Bone Formation Markers

Plasma bone alkaline phosphatase (bAP) is more sensitive than iPTH, total alkaline phosphatase, osteoccalcin (OC) and osteonectin to evaluate the bone remodeling in CKD patients [120, 124]. In dialysis patients, plasma bAP value not only provide useful information about bone formation rate, and but also estimate the type of bone disease. Serum bAP higher than 20ng/ml may predicts high bone turnover (with an 84% positive predictive value), whereas bAP concentration lower than 12.9ng/ml associates with low bone turnover (with a 72% positive predictive value) [124]. It is not clear whether it may separate adynamic bone disease patients from normal bone turnover individuals. Osteocalcin, a matrix protein, is now interesting for its role in bone formation. Despite it has been considered to be a marker for rate of bone formation, its role in ROD is still unclear. Further developments are necessary for other bone formation markers to be used clinically.

Conclusion

Bone mineral density (BMD) is reflective of changes in bone quantity, and thus can be used as a marker to assess the severity of osteoporosis. However, evaluation of fracture risk in patients with chronic kidney disease requires assessment of bone quality and changes in cortical bone, which cannot be detected with BMD measurements by dual-energy x-ray absorptiometry (DEXA) scan. Trans-iliac crest bone biopsy is the gold standard for characterizing changes in bone quality; however, the biopsy procedure is invasive and time consuming. For this reason, measurements of serum bone markers are used as additional non-invasive methods for monitoring bone quality.

Due to the unique pathophysiology of CKD-MBD, its management strategies are distinct from the treatment used in other types of osteoporosis. The cornerstone of management of CKD-MBD is to maintain normal bone turnover by maintaining adequate PTH and vitamin D receptor agonism. Normalizing phosphorous, calcium, calcitriol, and PTH levels is paramount, and is often therapeutically accomplished with the use of phosphate binders, vitamin D analogs, and calcimimetics.

References

[1] Clarke B. Normal bone anatomy and physiology. *Clin J Am Soc Nephrol* 2008;3 Suppl 3: S131-9.

[2] Avbersek-Luznik I, Balon BP, Rus I, Marc J. Increased bone resorption in HD patients: is it caused by elevated RANKL synthesis? *Nephrol Dial Transplant* 2005;20: 566-70.

[3] Ritz E, Stefanski A, Rambausek M. The role of the parathyroid glands in the uremic syndrome. *Am J Kidney Dis* 1995;26: 808-13.

[4] Rostand SG, Drueke TB. Parathyroid hormone, vitamin D, and cardiovascular disease in chronic renal failure. *Kidney Int* 1999;56: 383-92.

[5] Smith JC, Page MD, John R, Wheeler MH, Cockcroft JR, Scanlon MF, Davies JS. Augmentation of central arterial pressure in mild primary hyperparathyroidism. *J Clin Endocrinol Metab* 2000;85: 3515-9.

[6] Block GA, Klassen PS, Lazarus JM, Ofsthun N, Lowrie EG, Chertow GM. Mineral metabolism, mortality, and morbidity in maintenance hemodialysis. *J Am Soc Nephrol* 2004;15: 2208-18.

[7] Moorthi RN, Moe SM. CKD-mineral and bone disorder: core curriculum 2011. *Am J Kidney Dis* 2011;58: 1022-36.

[8] Miller PD. Diagnosis and treatment of osteoporosis in chronic renal disease. *Semin Nephrol* 2009;29: 144-55.

[9] Miller PD. Fragility fractures in chronic kidney disease: an opinion-based approach. *Cleve Clin J Med* 2009;76: 715-23.

[10] K/DOQI clinical practice guidelines for chronic kidney disease: evaluation, classification, and stratification. *Am J Kidney Dis* 2002;39: S1-266.

[11] Jamal SA, Gilbert J, Gordon C, Bauer DC. Cortical pQCT measures are associated with fractures in dialysis patients. *J Bone Miner Res* 2006;21: 543-8.

[12] Sakhaee K, Gonzalez GB. Update on renal osteodystrophy: pathogenesis and clinical management. *Am J Med Sci* 1999;317: 251-60.

[13] Huang GS, Chu TS, Lou MF, Hwang SL, Yang RS. Factors associated with low bone mass in the hemodialysis patients--a cross-sectional correlation study. *BMC Musculoskelet Disord* 2009;10: 60.

[14] Nickolas TL, McMahon DJ, Shane E. Relationship between moderate to severe kidney disease and hip fracture in the United States. *J Am Soc Nephrol* 2006;17: 3223-32.

[15] Ensrud KE, Lui LY, Taylor BC, Ishani A, Shlipak MG, Stone KL, Cauley JA, Jamal SA, Antoniucci DM, Cummings SR. Renal function and risk of hip and vertebral fractures in older women. *Arch Intern Med* 2007;167: 133-9.

[16] Dukas LC, Schacht E, Mazor Z, Stahelin HB. A new significant and independent risk factor for falls in elderly men and women: a low creatinine clearance of less than 65 ml/min. *Osteoporos Int* 2005;16: 332-8.

[17] Alem AM, Sherrard DJ, Gillen DL, Weiss NS, Beresford SA, Heckbert SR, Wong C, Stehman-Breen C. Increased risk of hip fracture among patients with end-stage renal disease. *Kidney Int* 2000;58: 396-9.

[18] Coco M, Rush H. Increased incidence of hip fractures in dialysis patients with low serum parathyroid hormone. *Am J Kidney Dis* 2000;36: 1115-21.

[19] Moe S, Drueke T, Cunningham J, Goodman W, Martin K, Olgaard K, Ott S, Sprague S, Lameire N, Eknoyan G. Definition, evaluation, and classification of renal osteodystrophy: a position statement from Kidney Disease: Improving Global Outcomes (KDIGO). *Kidney Int* 2006;69: 1945-53.

[20] Spasovski G, Zdravkovska V, Zabzun M, Antarorov R, Ivanovski K, Janakievska P, Neskovski J, Karceva-Sarajlia E, Panova B, Petrovska T, Zulbeari L, Masin-Spasovska J, Taleska-Matovska N, Gelev S. Achievements in CKD-MBD guidelines targets: is there a progress in the implementation practice? *Int Urol Nephrol* 2011.

[21] Moe SM, Radcliffe JS, White KE, Gattone VH, 2nd, Seifert MF, Chen X, Aldridge B, Chen NX. The pathophysiology of early-stage chronic kidney disease-mineral bone disorder (CKD-MBD) and response to phosphate binders in the rat. *J Bone Miner Res* 2011;26: 2672-81.

[22] Ward F, Watson A, Holian J. Chronic kidney disease-mineral bone disorder (CKD-MBD) management and associated cost in an Irish haemodialysis cohort. *Nephrol Dial Transplant* 2011;26: 3417.

[23] Midtby M, Magnus JH, Joakimsen RM. The Tromso Study: a population-based study on the variation in bone formation markers with

age, gender, anthropometry and season in both men and women. *Osteoporos Int* 2001;12: 835-43.
[24] Spaulding CM, Young G. Osteitis fibrosa cystica and chronic renal failure. *J Am Podiatr Med Assoc* 1997;87: 238-40.
[25] Jevtic V. Imaging of renal osteodystrophy. *Eur J Radiol* 2003;46: 85-95.
[26] Gavelli G, Zompatori M. Thoracic complications in uremic patients and in patients undergoing dialytic treatment: state of the art. *Eur Radiol* 1997;7: 708-17.
[27] Wittenberg A. The rugger jersey spine sign. *Radiology* 2004;230: 491-2.
[28] Fineman I, Johnson JP, Di-Patre PL, Sandhu H. Chronic renal failure causing brown tumors and myelopathy. Case report and review of pathophysiology and treatment. *J Neurosurg* 1999;90: 242-6.
[29] Leal CT, Lacativa PG, Gomes EM, Nunes RC, Costa FL, Gandelmann IH, Cavalcante MA, Farias ML. Surgical approach and clinical outcome of a deforming brown tumor at the maxilla in a patient with secondary hyperparathyroidism due to chronic renal failure. *Arq Bras Endocrinol Metabol* 2006;50: 963-7.
[30] Ix JH, Quarles LD, Chertow GM. Guidelines for disorders of mineral metabolism and secondary hyperparathyroidism should not yet be modified. *Nat Clin Pract Nephrol* 2006;2: 337-9.
[31] Baums MH, Klinger HM, Otte S. Morbus Teutschlander - a massive soft-tissue calcification of the foot in a patient on long-term hemodialysis. *Arch Orthop Trauma Surg* 2003;123: 51-3.
[32] Drueke TB. A clinical approach to the uraemic patient with extraskeletal calcifications. *Nephrol Dial Transplant* 1996;11 Suppl 3: 37-42.
[33] Monier-Faugere MC, Malluche HH. Trends in renal osteodystrophy: a survey from 1983 to 1995 in a total of 2248 patients. *Nephrol Dial Transplant* 1996;11 Suppl 3: 111-20.
[34] Coen G, Manni M, Addari O, Ballanti P, Pasquali M, Chicca S, Mazzaferro S, Napoletano I, Sardella D, Bonucci E. Metabolic acidosis and osteodystrophic bone disease in predialysis chronic renal failure: effect of calcitriol treatment. *Miner Electrolyte Metab* 1995;21: 375-82.
[35] Cannata-Andia JB. Hypokinetic azotemic osteodystrophy. *Kidney Int* 1998;54: 1000-16.
[36] Frazao JM, Martins P. Adynamic bone disease: clinical and therapeutic implications. *Curr Opin Nephrol Hypertens* 2009;18: 303-7.
[37] Stubbs JR, Liu S, Tang W, Zhou J, Wang Y, Yao X, Quarles LD. Role of hyperphosphatemia and 1,25-dihydroxyvitamin D in vascular

calcification and mortality in fibroblastic growth factor 23 null mice. *J Am Soc Nephrol* 2007;18: 2116-24.

[38] Galitzer H, Ben-Dov IZ, Silver J, Naveh-Many T. Parathyroid cell resistance to fibroblast growth factor 23 in secondary hyperparathyroidism of chronic kidney disease. *Kidney Int* 2010;77: 211-8.

[39] Hesse M, Frohlich LF, Zeitz U, Lanske B, Erben RG. Ablation of vitamin D signaling rescues bone, mineral, and glucose homeostasis in Fgf-23 deficient mice. *Matrix Biol* 2007;26: 75-84.

[40] Tsujikawa H, Kurotaki Y, Fujimori T, Fukuda K, Nabeshima Y. Klotho, a gene related to a syndrome resembling human premature aging, functions in a negative regulatory circuit of vitamin D endocrine system. *Mol Endocrinol* 2003;17: 2393-403.

[41] Gutierrez O, Isakova T, Rhee E, Shah A, Holmes J, Collerone G, Juppner H, Wolf M. Fibroblast growth factor-23 mitigates hyperphosphatemia but accentuates calcitriol deficiency in chronic kidney disease. *J Am Soc Nephrol* 2005;16: 2205-15.

[42] Bai X, Miao D, Li J, Goltzman D, Karaplis AC. Transgenic mice overexpressing human fibroblast growth factor 23 (R176Q) delineate a putative role for parathyroid hormone in renal phosphate wasting disorders. *Endocrinology* 2004;145: 5269-79.

[43] Oliveira RB, Cancela AL, Graciolli FG, Dos Reis LM, Draibe SA, Cuppari L, Carvalho AB, Jorgetti V, Canziani ME, Moyses RM. Early control of PTH and FGF23 in normophosphatemic CKD patients: a new target in CKD-MBD therapy? *Clin J Am Soc Nephrol* 2010;5: 286-91.

[44] Hasegawa H, Nagano N, Urakawa I, Yamazaki Y, Iijima K, Fujita T, Yamashita T, Fukumoto S, Shimada T. Direct evidence for a causative role of FGF23 in the abnormal renal phosphate handling and vitamin D metabolism in rats with early-stage chronic kidney disease. *Kidney Int* 2010;78: 975-80.

[45] Slatopolsky E, Robson AM, Elkan I, Bricker NS. Control of phosphate excretion in uremic man. J Clin Invest 1968;47: 1865-74.

[46] Goodman WG, Quarles LD. Development and progression of secondary hyperparathyroidism in chronic kidney disease: lessons from molecular genetics. *Kidney Int* 2008;74: 276-88.

[47] Martin DR, Ritter CS, Slatopolsky E, Brown AJ. Acute regulation of parathyroid hormone by dietary phosphate. Am J Physiol Endocrinol Metab 2005;289: E729-34.

[48] Davies MR, Lund RJ, Mathew S, Hruska KA. Low turnover osteodystrophy and vascular calcification are amenable to skeletal anabolism in an animal model of chronic kidney disease and the metabolic syndrome. *J Am Soc Nephrol* 2005;16: 917-28.
[49] Hruska KA, Mathew S. The roles of the skeleton and phosphorus in the CKD mineral bone disorder. *Adv Chronic Kidney Dis* 2011;18: 98-104.
[50] Lemann J, Jr., Litzow JR, Lennon EJ. The effects of chronic acid loads in normal man: further evidence for the participation of bone mineral in the defense against chronic metabolic acidosis. *J Clin Invest* 1966;45: 1608-14.
[51] Malluche HH, Ritz E, Lange HP, Kutschera L, Hodgson M, Seiffert U, Schoeppe W. Bone histology in incipient and advanced renal failure. *Kidney Int* 1976;9: 355-62.
[52] Rix M, Andreassen H, Eskildsen P, Langdahl B, Olgaard K. Bone mineral density and biochemical markers of bone turnover in patients with predialysis chronic renal failure. *Kidney Int* 1999;56: 1084-93.
[53] Yendt ER, Cohanim M, Jarzylo S, Jones G, Rosenberg G. Reduced creatinine clearance in primary osteoporosis in women. *J Bone Miner Res* 1993;8: 1045-52.
[54] Jones CA, McQuillan GM, Kusek JW, Eberhardt MS, Herman WH, Coresh J, Salive M, Jones CP, Agodoa LY. Serum creatinine levels in the US population: third National Health and Nutrition Examination Survey. *Am J Kidney Dis* 1998;32: 992-9.
[55] Schoppet M, Shroff RC, Hofbauer LC, Shanahan CM. Exploring the biology of vascular calcification in chronic kidney disease: what's circulating? *Kidney Int* 2008;73: 384-90.
[56] Demer LL, Tintut Y. Vascular calcification: pathobiology of a multifaceted disease. *Circulation* 2008;117: 2938-48.
[57] Wu-Wong JR, Nakane M, Ma J, Ruan X, Kroeger PE. Elevated phosphorus modulates vitamin D receptor-mediated gene expression in human vascular smooth muscle cells. *Am J Physiol Renal Physiol* 2007;293: F1592-604.
[58] Di Benedetto A, Marcelli D, D'Andrea A, Cice G, D'Isa S, Cappabianca F, Pacchiano G, D'Amato R, Oggero AR, Bonanno D, Pergamo O, Calabro R. Risk factors and underlying cardiovascular diseases in incident ESRD patients. *J Nephrol* 2005;18: 592-8.
[59] Mazzaferro S, Coen G, Bandini S, Borgatti PP, Ciaccheri M, Diacinti D, Ferranti E, Lusenti T, Mancini G, Monducci I, et al. Role of ageing,

chronic renal failure and dialysis in the calcification of mitral annulus. *Nephrol Dial Transplant* 1993;8: 335-40.

[60] Ritz E, Krempien B, Mehls O, Malluche H. Skeletal abnormalities in chronic renal insufficiency before and during maintenance hemodialysis. *Kidney Int* 1973;4: 116-27.

[61] Ritz E, Malluche HH, Roher HD, Krempien B, Koch KM, Andrassy K. [Some topical problems of subtotal parathyroidectomy in patients on haemodialysis]. D*tsch Med Wochenschr* 1973;98: 484-96.

[62] Di Leo C, Gallieni M, Bestetti A, Tagliabue L, Cozzolino M, Carpani P, Pozzato C, Tarolo GL, Brancaccio D. Cardiac and pulmonary calcification in a hemodialysis patient: partial regression 4 years after parathyroidectomy. *Clin Nephrol* 2003;59: 59-63.

[63] Zouboulis CC, Blume-Peytavi U, Lennert T, Stavropoulos PG, Schwarz A, Runkel N, Trautmann C, Orfanos CE. Fulminant metastatic calcinosis with cutaneous necrosis in a child with end-stage renal disease and tertiary hyperparathyroidism. *Br J Dermatol* 1996;135: 617-22.

[64] London GM, Marty C, Marchais SJ, Guerin AP, Metivier F, de Vernejoul MC. Arterial calcifications and bone histomorphometry in end-stage renal disease. *J Am Soc Nephrol* 2004;15: 1943-51.

[65] Asci G, Ok E, Savas R, Ozkahya M, Duman S, Toz H, Kayikcioglu M, Branscum AJ, Monier-Faugere MC, Herberth J, Malluche HH. The link between bone and coronary calcifications in CKD-5 patients on haemodialysis. *Nephrol Dial Transplant* 2011;26: 1010-5.

[66] Adragao T, Herberth J, Monier-Faugere MC, Branscum AJ, Ferreira A, Frazao JM, Dias Curto J, Malluche HH. Low bone volume--a risk factor for coronary calcifications in hemodialysis patients. *Clin J Am Soc Nephrol* 2009;4: 450-5.

[67] Schulz E, Arfai K, Liu X, Sayre J, Gilsanz V. Aortic calcification and the risk of osteoporosis and fractures. *J Clin Endocrinol Metab* 2004;89: 4246-53.

[68] Andress DL, Kopp JB, Maloney NA, Coburn JW, Sherrard DJ. Early deposition of aluminum in bone in diabetic patients on hemodialysis. *N Engl J Med* 1987;316: 292-6.

[69] Pei Y, Hercz G, Greenwood C, Segre G, Manuel A, Saiphoo C, Fenton S, Sherrard D. Renal osteodystrophy in diabetic patients. *Kidney Int* 1993;44: 159-64.

[70] Vincenti F, Arnaud SB, Recker R, Genant H, Amend WJ, Jr., Feduska NJ, Salvatierra O, Jr. Parathyroid and bone response of the diabetic patient to uremia. *Kidney Int* 1984;25: 677-82.

[71] Bouillon R. Diabetic bone disease. Low turnover osteoporosis related to decreased IGF-I production. *Verh K Acad Geneeskd Belg* 1992;54: 365-91; discussion 391-2.

[72] Bouillon R. Diabetic bone disease. *Calcif Tissue Int* 1991;49: 155-60.

[73] Cundy TF, Humphreys S, Watkins PJ, Parsons V. Hyperparathyroid bone disease in diabetic renal failure. *Diabetes Res* 1990;14: 191-6.

[74] Yamaguchi T, Sugimoto T. Bone metabolism and fracture risk in type 2 diabetes mellitus [Review]. *Endocr J* 2011;58: 613-24.

[75] Montagnani A, Gonnelli S, Alessandri M, Nuti R. Osteoporosis and risk of fracture in patients with diabetes: an update. Aging *Clin Exp Res* 2011;23: 84-90.

[76] Betteridge DJ. Thiazolidinediones and fracture risk in patients with Type 2 diabetes. *Diabet* Med 2011;28: 759-71.

[77] Schwartz AV, Vittinghoff E, Bauer DC, Hillier TA, Strotmeyer ES, Ensrud KE, Donaldson MG, Cauley JA, Harris TB, Koster A, Womack CR, Palermo L, Black DM. Association of BMD and FRAX score with risk of fracture in older adults with type 2 diabetes. *JAMA* 2011;305: 2184-92.

[78] Szulc P, Varennes A, Delmas PD, Goudable J, Chapurlat R. Men with metabolic syndrome have lower bone mineral density but lower fracture risk--the MINOS study. *J Bone Miner Res* 2010;25: 1446-54.

[79] Boyanov M, Bakalov D, Boneva Z. Bone mineral density in men with and without the metabolic syndrome. *Aging Male* 2009;12: 62-5.

[80] Grzegorzewska AE, Mlot-Michalska M. Low molecular weight heparins and antiplatelet drugs, and bone mineral density in dialysis patients. *Adv Perit Dial* 2008;24: 125-31.

[81] Drueke TB. Abnormal skeletal response to parathyroid hormone and the expression of its receptor in chronic uremia. *Pediatr Nephrol* 1996;10: 348-50.

[82] Matuszkiewicz-Rowinska J, Skorzewska K, Radowicki S, Sokalski A, Przedlacki J, Niemczyk S, Wlodarczyk D, Puka J, Switalski M. The benefits of hormone replacement therapy in pre-menopausal women with oestrogen deficiency on haemodialysis. *Nephrol Dial Transplant* 1999;14: 1238-43.

[83] Sugiya N, Nakashima A, Takasugi N, Kawai A, Kiribayashi K, Tanaka J, Kohno N, Yorioka N. Endogenous estrogen may prevent bone loss in

postmenopausal hemodialysis patients throughout life. *Osteoporos Int* 2011;22: 1573-9.

[84] Bouchard J, Ouimet D, Vallee M, Lafrance JP, Leblanc M, Senecal L, Bonnardeaux A, Mathieu JP, Pichette V. Comparison of the prevalence of calcidiol insufficiency in predialysis and osteoporotic populations. Int Urol Nephrol 2009;41: 983-8.

[85] Heinonen A, Oja P, Kannus P, Sievanen H, Haapasalo H, Manttari A, Vuori I. Bone mineral density in female athletes representing sports with different loading characteristics of the skeleton. *Bone* 1995;17: 197-203.

[86] Yamazaki S, Ichimura S, Iwamoto J, Takeda T, Toyama Y. Effect of walking exercise on bone metabolism in postmenopausal women with osteopenia/osteoporosis. J *Bone Miner Metab* 2004;22: 500-8.

[87] Ubara Y, Tagami T, Nakanishi S, Sawa N, Hoshino J, Suwabe T, Katori H, Takemoto F, Hara S, Takaichi K. Significance of minimodeling in dialysis patients with adynamic bone disease. *Kidney Int* 2005;68: 833-9.

[88] Spindler A, Paz S, Berman A, Lucero E, Contino N, Penalba A, Tirado S, Santana M, Zeballos AC. Muscular strength and bone mineral density in haemodialysis patients. *Nephrol Dial Transplant* 1997;12: 128-32.

[89] Chamay A, Tschantz P. Mechanical influences in bone remodeling. Experimental research on Wolff's law. *J Biomech* 1972;5: 173-80.

[90] Bianchi ML, Colantonio G, Montesano A, Trevisan C, Ortolani S, Rossi R, Buccianti G. Bone mass status in different degrees of chronic renal failure. *Bone* 1992;13: 225-8.

[91] Heaf JG, Nielsen LP, Mogensen NB. Use of bone mineral content determination in the evaluation of osteodystrophy among hemodialysis patients. *Nephron* 1983;35: 103-7.

[92] Eeckhout E, Verbeelen D, Sennesael J, Kaufman L, Jonckheer MH. Monitoring of bone mineral content in patients on regular hemodialysis. Nephron 1989;52: 158-61.

[93] Petrauskiene V, Bumblyte IA, Sileikiene E, Gineikaite R, Burbulyte R. [Evaluation of bone mineral density and its importance for hemodialysis patients]. Medicina (Kaunas) 2007;43 Suppl 1: 90-5.

[94] Atsumi K, Kushida K, Yamazaki K, Shimizu S, Ohmura A, Inoue T. Risk factors for vertebral fractures in renal osteodystrophy. *Am J Kidney Dis* 1999;33: 287-93.

[95] Barreto FC, Barreto DV, Moyses RM, Neves CL, Jorgetti V, Draibe SA, Canziani ME, Carvalho AB. Osteoporosis in hemodialysis patients

revisited by bone histomorphometry: a new insight into an old problem. *Kidney Int* 2006;69: 1852-7.

[96] Dimkovic N, Oreopoulos DG. High and low turnover bone disease in patients on chronic peritoneal dialysis. Nephrol Dial Transplant 2001;16 *Suppl* 6: 114-6.

[97] Spasovski GB, Bervoets AR, Behets GJ, Ivanovski N, Sikole A, Dams G, Couttenye MM, De Broe ME, D'Haese PC. Spectrum of renal bone disease in end-stage renal failure patients not yet on dialysis. Nephrol Dial Transplant 2003;18: 1159-66.

[98] Sherrard DJ, Hercz G, Pei Y, Maloney NA, Greenwood C, Manuel A, Saiphoo C, Fenton SS, Segre GV. The spectrum of bone disease in end-stage renal failure--an evolving disorder. *Kidney Int* 1993;43: 436-42.

[99] Grzegorzewska AE, Mlot-Michalska M. Bone mineral density, its predictors, and outcomes in peritoneal dialysis patients. *Adv Perit Dial* 2011;27: 140-5.

[100] Ersoy FF, Passadakis SP, Tam P, Memmos ED, Katopodis PK, Ozener C, Akcicek F, Camsari T, Ates K, Ataman R, Vlachojannis JG, Dombros AN, Utas C, Akpolat T, Bozfakioglu S, Wu G, Karayaylali I, Arinsoy T, Stathakis PC, Yavuz M, Tsakiris JD, Dimitriades CA, Yilmaz ME, Gultekin M, Karayalcin B, Yardimsever M, Oreopoulos DG. Bone mineral density and its correlation with clinical and laboratory factors in chronic peritoneal dialysis patients. *J Bone Miner Metab* 2006;24: 79-86.

[101] Jeong JU, Lee HK, Kim YJ, Kim JS, Kang SS, Kim SB. Nutritional markers, not markers of bone turnover, are related predictors of bone mineral density in chronic peritoneal dialysis patients. *Clin Nephrol* 2010;74: 336-42.

[102] Lu KC, Ma WY, Yu JC, Wu CC, Chu P. Bone Turnover Markers Predict Changes in Bone Mineral Density after Parathyroidectomy in Patients with Renal Hyperparathyroidism. *Clin Endocrinol (Oxf)* 2012; 76: 634–642.

[103] Salusky IB, Goodman WG, Sahney S, Gales B, Perilloux A, Wang HJ, Elashoff RM, Juppner H. Sevelamer controls parathyroid hormone-induced bone disease as efficiently as calcium carbonate without increasing serum calcium levels during therapy with active vitamin D sterols. *J Am Soc Nephrol* 2005;16: 2501-8.

[104] Wu CC, Chang JH, Chen CC, Su SB, Yang LK, Ma WY, Zheng CM, Diang LK, Lu KC. Calcitriol treatment attenuates inflammation and

oxidative stress in hemodialysis patients with secondary hyperparathyroidism. *Tohoku J Exp Med* 2011;223: 153-9.

[105] Zheng CM, Chu P, Wu CC, Ma WY, Hung KC, Hsu YH, Lin YF, Diang LK, Lu KC. Association between increased serum osteoprotegerin levels and improvement in bone mineral density after parathyroidectomy in hemodialysis patients. *Tohoku J* Exp Med 2012;226: 19-27.

[106] Spasovski GB. Bone biopsy as a diagnostic tool in the assessment of renal osteodystrophy. *Int J Artif Organs* 2004;27: 918-23.

[107] Andress DL. Adynamic bone in patients with chronic kidney disease. *Kidney Int* 2008;73: 1345-54.

[108] Hernandez D, Concepcion MT, Lorenzo V, Martinez ME, Rodriguez A, De Bonis E, Gonzalez-Posada JM, Felsenfeld AJ, Rodriguez M, Torres A. Adynamic bone disease with negative aluminium staining in predialysis patients: prevalence and evolution after maintenance dialysis. *Nephrol Dial Transplant* 1994;9: 517-23.

[109] Sugimoto T, Ritter C, Morrissey J, Hayes C, Slatopolsky E. Effects of high concentrations of glucose on PTH secretion in parathyroid cells. *Kidney Int* 1990;37: 1522-7.

[110] Piraino B, Chen T, Cooperstein L, Segre G, Puschett J. Fractures and vertebral bone mineral density in patients with renal osteodystrophy. *Clin Nephrol* 1988;30: 57-62.

[111] Mawad HW, Sawaya BP, Sarin R, Malluche HH. Calcific uremic arteriolopathy in association with low turnover uremic bone disease. *Clin Nephrol* 1999;52: 160-6.

[112] Avram MM, Mittman N, Myint MM, Fein P. Importance of low serum intact parathyroid hormone as a predictor of mortality in hemodialysis and peritoneal dialysis patients: 14 years of prospective observation. *Am J Kidney Dis* 2001;38: 1351-7.

[113] Fujimori A, Yorifuji M, Sakai M, Oyama M, Nakao N, Tokuyama M, Fukagawa M. Low-calcium dialysate improves mineral metabolism in hemodialysis patients. *Clin Nephrol* 2007;67: 20-4.

[114] Holgado R, Haire H, Ross D, Sprague S, Pahl M, Jara A, Martin-Malo A, Rodriguez M, Almaden Y, Felsenfeld AJ. Effect of a low calcium dialysate on parathyroid hormone secretion in diabetic patients on maintenance hemodialysis. *J Bone Miner Res* 2000;15: 927-35.

[115] Unal A, Kocyigit I, Sipahioglu MH, Tokgoz B, Kavuncuoglu F, Oymak O, Utas C. Loss of bone mineral density in renal transplantation recipients. *Transplant Proc* 2010;42: 3550-3.

[116] Rolla D, Ballanti P, Marsano L, Bianchi G, Messa P, Paoletti E, Cannella G. Bone disease in long-term renal transplant recipients with severe osteopenia: a cross-sectional study. *Transplantation* 2006;81: 915-21.

[117] Weber TJ, Quarles LD. Preventing bone loss after renal transplantation with bisphosphonates: we can... but should we? *Kidney Int* 2000;57: 735-7.

[118] Nuttall ME, Patton AJ, Olivera DL, Nadeau DP, Gowen M. Human trabecular bone cells are able to express both osteoblastic and adipocytic phenotype: implications for osteopenic disorders. *J Bone Miner Res* 1998;13: 371-82.

[119] Monier-Faugere MC, Mawad H, Qi Q, Friedler RM, Malluche HH. High prevalence of low bone turnover and occurrence of osteomalacia after kidney transplantation. *J Am Soc Nephrol* 2000;11: 1093-9.

[120] Urena P, De Vernejoul MC. Circulating biochemical markers of bone remodeling in uremic patients. *Kidney Int* 1999;55: 2141-56.

[121] Fujimori A, Okada S, Sakai M, Tome K, Fukagawa M. Relationship between biochemical markers and radial cortical bone changes in hemodialysis patients. Nephron Clin Pract 2011;118: c375-9.

[122] Tolouian R, Hernandez GT, Chiang WY, Gupta A. A new approach for evaluating bone turnover in chronic kidney disease. *Eur J Intern Med* 2010;21: 230-2.

[123] Cejka D, Jager-Lansky A, Kieweg H, Weber M, Bieglmayer C, Haider DG, Diarra D, Patsch JM, Kainberger F, Bohle B, Haas M. Sclerostin serum levels correlate positively with bone mineral density and microarchitecture in haemodialysis patients. *Nephrol Dial Transplant* 2012;27: 226-30.

[124] Urena, P. Hruby, M. Ferreira, A. Ang, K. S. de Vernejoul, M. C. Plasma total versus bone alkaline phosphatase as markers of bone turnover in hemodialysis patients. J Am Soc Nephrol 1996;7(3):506-12.

In: Bone Loss
Editor: Kuo-Cheng Lu
ISBN: 978-1-62417-169-7

Chapter 2

OSTEOPOROSIS AND DIABETES

***Chang-Hsun Hsieh*[1] *and Dee-Pei*[2]**

[1]Division of Endocrinology and Metabolism, Department of Internal Medicine, Tri-Service General Hospital, National Defense Medical Center, Taipei, Taiwan

[2]Division of Endocrinology and Metabolism, Department of Internal Medicine, Cardinal Tien Hospital, School of Medicine, Fu Jen Catholic University, New Taipei City, Taiwan

ABSTRACT

There is a growing body of evidence that diabetes mellitus (DM) and osteoporosis are closely bound together. Both diseases are increasing in prevalence rate with aging, being often silent in the early stage of the disease and sharing the similar predisposing factors. Co-existence of both diseases will increase personal and social-economic burden, therefore, preventive strategies toward both disorders is needed. The interaction between DM and osteoporosis is complex and different in varying types of DM. Recent meta-analysis had confirmed that both type 1 and type 2 diabetes are associated with increasing risk of bone fracture. However, the bone mineral density is decreased, normal or increased in subjects of type 1 diabetes and type 2 diabetes, respectively. The mechanisms of osteoporosis in DM are complex, involving the process of both bone strength and bone quality. The physician should be aware of the risk factors of osteoporosis and extensively evaluated before starting the management of osteoporosis in subjects with DM. The treatment of osteoporosis is similar to non-diabetics, which included both non-pharmacological and pharmacological intervention. Currently, there is no formal clinical recommendation in managing osteoporosis in subjects of DM. It needs more clinical evidence with a focus on patients with DM to provide more information to establish the guideline of the treatment of osteoporosis in subjects of DM.

INTRODUCTION

Osteoporosis is the thinning of bone tissue and loss of bone density that mainly affects the elderly, especially postmenopausal females. The disease is characterized by a decrease in bone mineral density (BMD) and quality, microarchitectural deterioration, and mineralization of bone tissues, subsequently leading to increased bone fragility and risk of bone fracture [1]. Like other chronic disorders, it is progressive and can result in significant co-morbidity and mortality as well as increased social and economic burdens. Osteoporosis is etiologically multifactorial and has been divided into primary and secondary causes. Primary osteoporosis is diagnosed when a secondary cause cannot be identified and is further divided into type I, which occurs in postmenopausal females because of estrogen deficiency, and type II (also called senile type), which often occurs in the elderly because of calcium deficiency and aging. There is increasing evidence suggesting that diabetes mellitus (DM) and osteoporosis are closely associated. Both diseases are increasing in prevalence because of aging and are often silent during the early disease stages, but share similar predisposing factors. The prevalence of osteoporosis in patients with diabetes depends on the type and duration of diabetes and gender. The increasing number of patients with DM and osteoporosis will probably continue to increase the burden of health cost. Therefore, it is warranted to provide adequate information and develop a strategy for early detection and prevention of both diseases.

The association between diabetes and osteoporosis is complex and remains largely unclear because osteoporosis may be a complication of diabetes, or diabetes may be a risk factor for osteoporosis, or both. However, several endocrine disorders such as Cushing syndrome and hyperthyroidism can cause not only secondary diabetes but also secondary osteoporosis, which further confounds the association [2]. Traditionally, osteoporosis has not been considered a chronic complication of diabetes. However, several bone disorders can develop in patients with diabetes, and osteoporosis is the most patients met the criteria for osteoporosis (T-value ≤ −2.5 SD). A study conducted by López-Ibarra et al. measured BMD at the time of T1D diagnosis at the lumbar spine and femoral neck in 32 patients (22 males and 10 females and age, 20–39 years)[19]. The authors noted that BMD in patients with T1D at the time of diagnosis was lower than that in non-diabetic controls. This finding suggested that osteoporosis should not be considered a complication of DM, which is contrary to previous studies.

Similarly, decreased BMD was noted in young patients with T1D. Gunczler et al. measured BMD at the lumbar spine in 23 prepubertal children (median age, 9.5 years and median diabetes duration, 5.8 years) and found that BMD in patients with T1D was lower than that in non-diabetic controls [5]. When the lumbar spine Z-scores were analyzed, a significant difference was observed for BMD between patients with T1D diagnosed for <3 months and those diagnosed with DM ≥3 months. A study by Liu et al. compared BMD between 39 teenage (age, 13–19 years) and 33 post-teenage (age, 20–37 years) female patients with T1D and 91 female age-matched non-diabetic controls and found that BMD at the femoral neck in female patients aged >20 years was significantly lower than that in female patients aged <20 years and non-diabetic controls [9]. The authors concluded that female patients with DM exhibited BMD differences early in their diabetes status and BMD decreased during post-teenage years.

Nevertheless, few studies have documented that BMD did not decrease in patients with T1D [23-25]. Lunt et al. measured BMD at the femoral neck and lumbar spine in 99 female patients with DM (median age, 42 years and median diabetes duration, 27 years) and found no differences in BMD between pre- and postmenopausal female patients with DM and non-diabetic controls [24]. Rozadilla et al. measured BMD at the femoral neck and lumbar spine in 88 Spanish adults with T1D in the absence of obvious complications (mean age, 28.9 years and diabetes duration, 11.2 years) and found that BMD at the lumbar spine, but not at the femoral neck, was lower than that in non-diabetic controls [23]. The authors claimed that bone loss may not be a major problem in young patients with relative short-term T1D and without severe complications.

A recent meta-analysis by Vestergaard et al. concluded that BMD at the spine and hip in patients with DM was lower than that in non-diabetic controls [26]. Several recent studies have also revealed similar results. Mastrandrea conducted a 2-year prospective follow-up to determine the natural course of BMD in young patients with T1D [16]. A total of 63 female patients with T1D (age, 13–35 years) were enrolled in the study. He found that BMD in patients common. Several possible mechanisms associate diabetes with osteopo. but the mechanisms differ between diabetes types. An increasing average expectancy of patients with diabetes, accompanied by improvements medical care, has increased the significance of osteoporosis. Therefore, physicians should be aware of the epidemiology, risk factors, and underlying mechanisms of osteoporosis in patients with DM to provide adequate clinical recommendations. This chapter will discuss the current information available on the association between osteoporosis and diabetes.

1. Association between Diabetes and Osteoporosis

1.1. Type 1 Diabetes and Osteoporosis

The association between type 1 diabetes (T1D) and osteoporosis is complex. Although there are inconsistent findings, most studies have suggested that patients with T1D have decreased BMD, which is determined using the dual energy X-ray absorptiometry (DEXA) method. DEXA has been a worldwide used technique to define osteoporosis [3]. Decreases in BMD affect all ages, including children, adolescents [4-12], and adults [13-22].

Muñoz-Torres et al. measured BMD at the lumbar spine and proximal femur using DEXA in 94 patients with T1D (age, 20–56 years and diabetes duration, 1–35 years)[22]. Of the 94 patients, 18 (19.1%) met the diagnostic criteria for osteoporosis. Furthermore, the authors considered osteopenia as a complication in patients with T1D. Kayath et al. measured BMD at the lumbar spine and femoral region in 23 patients (age, 21–53 years and diabetes duration, 2.3–20 years)[21]. All patients had a second BMD measurement approximately 2 years later. The authors noted that BMD at the spine in patients with and without osteopenia was higher in the second evaluation than that at baseline. Nevertheless, BMD in patients with osteopenia was consistently lower than that in patients without osteopenia at the end of the study. However, no patients had their condition significantly worsened. The authors concluded that BMD in majority of patients with DM did not worsen rapidly. Kemink et al. measured BMD in 35 patients (median age, 37.6 years and diabetes duration, 8.5 years) and found that BMD in patients with T1D was lower than that in non-diabetic controls [20]. Osteopenia, defined by a T score (T-value ≤ -1 SD) of the femoral neck and/or the lumbar spine, was noted in 67% of male patients with diabetes and 57% of female patients with diabetes in this study. None of the female patients and 14% of the male with T1D was lower than that in non-diabetic controls, and the difference persisted over time. Heilman et al. (11) measured BMD at the lumbar spine in 30 children with inadequately controlled T1D (age, 4.7–18.6 years and mean diabetes duration, 5.4 years) and found that BMD in children with T1D was significantly lower than that in non-diabetic controls. However, these differences were mostly observed in male patients. A study by Saha et al. (12) compared BMD at the radius, tibia, lumbar spine, and proximal femur and bony structures between adolescents with T1D and non-diabetic controls by peripheral quantitative computed tomography (pQCT) and DEXA [12]. The authors suggested that T1D was associated with lower BMD, and diabetes-related abnormalities were predominant in male patients.

There are several patient characteristics that influence or can predict the association between T1D and osteoporosis. First, gender may influence the association between T1D and osteoporosis. Hamilton et al. found that osteoporosis was more common and BMD was lower in male patients with T1D than that in age-matched non-diabetic controls [25]. However, female patients with T1D and non-diabetic controls showed similar BMD. These results were compatible with a study that concluded that male patients with T1D had a higher prevalence of osteoporosis and osteopenia than female patients with T1D [20]. Another study observed that although BMD in patients with T1D was lower than those in patients with type 2 diabetes (T2D) in both genders, significant difference was found only in male patients after adjusting for age and body mass index (BMI) [18]. Hadjidakis et al. reported that age-adjusted BMD at the vertebrae was different between patients with T1D and non-diabetic controls [27]. But the difference was not significant in female patients. In a study involving 30 young children with short-term T1D (diabetes duration, 5.4 years) and inadequate glycemic control [mean glycosylated hemoglobin (HbA1c) level = 9.8%], BMD in patients with T1D was lower than that in non-diabetic controls, and this difference was attributed to the male patients. Gender differences were also observed in the previous mentioned studies [11,12]. The gender difference of BMD may although not fully explained, attributed to the sex hormones difference between genders.

Diabetes duration is a factor associated with BMD. Several studies suggested that BMD was negatively associated with diabetes duration (10,21,22). In contrast, other studies did not report this association (6,15,24,27). Many specialists claimed that diabetes duration influenced BMD merely as a consequence of the natural course of diabetes and did not actually influence BMD. Obesity is a typical clinical feature of DM (mainly T2D) that may play a role in increased BMD. Several studies confirmed that BMD was positively associated with obesity (mostly BMI) [22,24,25,28]. A meta-regression analysis showed that BMI was a major determinant for BMD at the hip and spine [26]. Age or age at diabetes onset was also associated with BMD. A negative association was noted between BMD and age in previous studies [6,10]. Liu et al. found that BMD at the femoral neck in female patients with T1D older than 20 years was higher than that in non-diabetic controls, but not in patients younger than 20 years [9]. A similar conclusion was drawn in another study, although statistically insignificant BMD in patients with DM younger than 20 years was higher than that in non-diabetic controls [16]. However, age at diabetes onset did not influence BMD in patients with T1D [27]. Furthermore, the presence and/or the severity of diabetic complications were associated with decreased BMD in patients with T1D [22-24], but this association has not been observed in other studies [15,28]. Adequate metabolic control was positively associated with BMD [8,17]; however, these results were not in agreement with other previous studies [6,15,16,19,20,21,28]. Furthermore, Vestergaard et al. found that the glycemic control index was not associated with BMD [26].

It is difficult to estimate the exact prevalence rate of osteoporosis in patients with T1D because of a lack of large-scale population studies, methods, and sites for BMD measurement. Based on previous studies using DEXA, 50%–60% of patients with T1D were diagnosed with osteopenia and 14%–20% with osteoporosis [20,29].

1.2. Type 2 Diabetes and Osteoporosis

Unlike patients with T1D, those with T2D have been found to benefit from the protective mechanisms of osteoporosis since BMD remained normal or increased, although BMD findings in patients with T2D were inconsistent in previous studies. However, most studies included females (especially, postmenopausal females) and small sample sizes. Thus, BMD in patients with T2D was higher than that in non-diabetic controls, although some showed no difference. Paradoxically, few studies have found decreased BMD in patients with T2D.

Based on the WHO definition of osteoporosis, van Daele et al. conducted a cross-sectional study involving 5931 patients (2481 males and 3450 females and age, >55 years) and found that patients with T2D had a 3% higher BMD than non-diabetic controls [30]. Several studies confirmed this finding [18,28, 31-43]. Barrett-Connor et al. surveyed a community-based population of older adults to examine the association of glucose tolerance with T2D and osteoporosis [31]. BMD was measured at the ultradistal wrist and midradius by single photon absorptiometry and at the femoral neck and lumbar spine by DEXA. Among the 627 patients (236 males and 391 females and mean age, 72 years), 41 male and 39 female patients had T2D, and 56 male and 110 female patients had impaired glucose tolerance (IGT). BMD in patients with T2D was higher than that in patients with normal glucose tolerance (NGT), but only in the female population. Kwon et al. measured BMD at the lumbar spine by DEXA in 185 patients with T2D and found that BMD in patients with T2D was higher than that in non-diabetic controls and bone loss related to menopause began before the onset of menopause [33]. Miedany et al. measured BMD at the lumbar spine by CT in 40 postmenopausal female patients and 20 males with T2D [34]. They found that BMD in female patients with T2D was higher than that in non-diabetic controls. Schwartz et al. analyzed 9654 female patients over the age of 65 years and determined that 657 of them had T2D onset after the age of 40 years [36]. They concluded that T2D was associated with increased BMD. Sert et al. conducted a prospective study involving a total of 277 patients with T2D (age, 30–60 years)[37]. BMD at the lumbar vertebrae and the femur was measured by DEXA and compared with that in 262 non-diabetic controls. BMD at the femoral neck increased among both genders with T2D aged 51–60 years. However, BMD showed a paradoxical decrease at the lumbar regions in male patients with T2D compared with non-diabetic controls in all age groups. The authors suggested that patients with T2D may have lower, similar, or higher BMD measurements, which may be influenced by age and anatomical region.

A population-based family study of 600 subjects from 34 Mexican–American families found that BMD at the hip in female patients with T2D was significantly higher than that in patients without T2D, which remained significantly different even after adjustment for age, BMI, and menopausal status [38]. Another large-scale population study, called the "The Health, Aging, and Body Composition Study," included 2979 elderly patients (age, 70–79 years), including 566 (19%) with T2D at baseline [39]. BMD at the spine was measured by CT and that at the hip was measured by DEXA and was higher in patients with T2D than in non-diabetic controls. Another cohort study, conducted by Dennison et al. involved a total of 465 male and 444 female subjects (age, 59–71 years) without previous T2D diagnoses [40]. Among them, 33 male and 32 female patients were diagnosed with T2D, and BMD in these newly diagnosed patients was higher than that in patients with NGT, with female patients predominating over male patients. Bonds et al.

analyzed data from the "Women's Health Initiative Observational Cohort," which was a prospective study of more than 90,000 postmenopausal female patients [42]. Analysis confirmed that BMD at the hip and spine in female patients with T2D was higher than that in non-diabetic controls. According to the latest analysis from the dataset of the three large-scale studies, "Study of Osteoporotic Fractures," "The Osteoporotic Fractures in Men Study," and "The Health, Aging, and Body Composition Study," patients with T2D had a higher T-score than those without T2D [44].

Two studies showed that BMD in patients with T2D did not differ from those without diabetes [45,46]. Sosa measured BMD by DEXA and pQCT in 47 patients with T2D [45]. However, no differences in BMD were found between patients with T2D and non-diabetic controls. Paradoxically, some studies observed that BMD in patients with T2D was lower than that in non-diabetic controls. Majima et al. enrolled 145 Japanese subjects with T2D (64 males and 81 females) and 95 age-matched non-diabetic controls (41 males and 54 females) [47]. BMD was measured at the lumbar spine, femoral neck, and distal radius by DEXA. BMD and Z-score at the distal radii were significantly lower in patients with T2D than those in non-diabetic controls. In Saudi Arabia, Al-Maatouq enrolled 104 postmenopausal female patients with T2D and 101 non-diabetic controls and found that decreased BMD was attributed to diabetes status [48]. A study by Sert et al. observed that BMD in male patients with T2D was lower at the lumbar region, but not at other anatomical locations [37]. However, a recent meta-analysis by Vestergaard et al. found that BMD increased in patients with T2D [26].

These discrepancies in BMD measurement in patients with T2D may be due to several factors. For instance, there was a gender bias for osteoporosis and T2D. Although many studies have shown that BMD in patients with T2D was higher than that in non-diabetic controls, the difference occurred mostly in the female population [31,34,40]. El Miedany et al. stated that gender differences may be explained by the occurrence of obesity and increased androgenicity reported in female patients with hyperglycemia and hyperinsulinemia [34]. Furthermore, the anatomical site of BMD measurement may partially account for this difference as well as the rate of bone loss. BMD decreased more rapidly at the hip of patients with T2D compared with non-diabetic controls. Nevertheless, the decrease in bone loss at the lumbar spine was relatively slower in females with T2D than in non-diabetic controls [43]. Furthermore, BMD positively associated with BMI [32], and insulin level [32,38] and negatively with age, menopausal age, and diabetes duration [33]. Inadequate glycemic control had a negative effect on BMD [47], but there was no association between BMD and HbA1c levels or the presence of chronic diabetic complications [28].

It is challenging to draw accurate conclusions from these studies because most were performed with a small study population. There is a latency period before the diagnosis of T2D; hence, diagnosis is often delayed for several years. Recently, the "Korea Rural Genomic Cohort Study" examined BMD in patients with IGT, but it was similar to that in non-diabetic controls [49].

2. Association between Diabetes and Bone Fracture

2.1. Type 1 Diabetes and Risk of Bone Fracture

It is reasonable to hypothesize that the risk of fracture increased because of its decreased BMD in patients with T1D. However, it was controversial whether decreased BMD influences the occurrence of bone fractures until recent studies confirmed a close association. "The Nord-Trøndelag Health Survey" was conducted to evaluate the occurrence of hip fractures in female patients with T1D [50]. A total of 35,444 patients (age, >50 years) were enrolled in the study and followed up for 9 years. The relative risk (RR) for hip fractures in female patients with T1D after adjusting for other risk factors was 6.9 compared to that in non-diabetic controls, but only the occurrence in females was statistically significant. Nicodemus et al. conducted a large prospective cohort involving over 32,000 postmenopausal female patients in Iowa and monitored them over a period of 11 years [51]. They found that patients with T1D had 12.25 times higher risk for developing further hip osteoporosis than patients without after adjusting for confounding factors. A population-based cohort study from the Swedish Inpatient Register involved a total of 24,605 patients with T1D (12,551 males and 12,054 females) under the age of 31 years who were monitored for hip fracture. The study found that the fracture risk increased in both genders having T1D [52]. A Danish case-control study involved a total of 124,655 patients with a fracture history and 373,962 sex- and aged-matched non-diabetic controls to examine fracture risk in patients with diabetes, and the impact of prescribing medication on relative fracture risk [53]. The authors concluded that T1D was associated with an increased fracture risk [odds ratio (OR) = 1.3 after adjustment for confounders] and increased risk for hip fractures (OR = 1.7). Furthermore,

T1D was associated with an increased risk of spine fractures (OR = 2.5). Janghorbani et al. drew similar conclusions from the "The Nurses' Health Study," which evaluated the potential risk factors for further hip fractures in 109,983 female patients (age, 34–59 years)[54]. He claimed that the age-adjusted RR of hip fracture in patients with T1D was 7.1 compared with that in patients without diabetes, and the risk was attenuated, but persisted, after controlling for other risk factors. The same author conducted a systemic review of 16 eligible studies involving 836,941 patients with T1D and found that T1D was associated with an increased risk of hip fracture with RR of 6.3 compared with that in non-diabetic controls [55]. Similar results were reported in another meta-analysis of 5 T1D studies, which found an increased risk of hip fractures with RR of 6.94 compared with that in patients without DM. The presence of diabetic complications may increase fracture risk [26].

2.2. Type 2 Diabetes and Risk of Bone Fracture

Unlike patients with T1D, those with T2D may have advantageous bone protection because BMD was normal or increased, although results have been inconsistent. Several studies have examined the association between increased bone fractures and T2D. "The Nord-Trøndelag Health Survey" evaluated hip fractures in female patients with T2D. After a 9-year follow-up period, RR of hip fracture in female patients with T2D (age, 50–74 years and diabetes duration, >5 years) was 1.8 compared with that in non-diabetic controls [50]. Furthermore, the RR was 1.5 after adjustment for medical factors related to T2D, but remained significantly higher than that in non-diabetic controls. Nicodemus et al. assessed postmenopausal female patients with T2D for fracture risk and found 490 hip fractures during a follow-up period of 306,900 person-years [51]. Female patients with T2D had a 1.7 times higher risk of hip fracture than non-diabetic controls. A higher fracture incidence was associated with longer diabetes duration and the use of any type of medication. Furthermore, patients with newly diagnosed T2D had a higher risk (RR = 1.6) of hip fracture than those with NGT during follow-up. Schwartz et al. analyzed data from a prospective study titled the "Study of Osteoporotic Features Research Group.", and found that patients with T2D were associated with a higher risk of bone fractures than non-diabetic controls [36]. Furthermore, female patients with T2D who were not using insulin had an increased risk of hip and proximal humerus fractures than non-diabetic controls after adjusting for other factors associated with fractures and diabetes. Conversely, those using insulin had more than double the risk of foot fractures than non-diabetic controls.

"The Blue Mountains Eye Study" was a prospective study that enrolled 3,654 patients with T2D (age, >49 years) who were monitored for 2 years to evaluate fracture risk and diabetes-related conditions [56]. Several diabetes-related factors were significantly associated with an increased risk of all fractures, including the presence of diabetic retinopathy, diabetes duration greater than 10 years, the presence of cataracts, and insulin treatment. A longitudinal study of 3050 Mexican–American patients (age, >65 years), including 690 with diabetes, were monitored for 7 years to evaluate the risk of hip fractures [57]. The study reported an increased frequency of hip fractures in patients with T2D compared to non-diabetic controls [hazard ratio (HR) = 1.57]. Furthermore, patients taking insulin had the higher risk than non-diabetic controls (HR = 2.84) after controlling for other variables. Vestergaard et al. found that T2D was associated with an increased risk of all fractures (OR = 1.2 after adjustment for confounders), especially hip fractures (OR = 1.4)[26]. Furthermore, T2D was associated with a significant increase in forearm fractures (OR = 1.2). However, the risk of spine fractures did not increase with T2D. Interestingly, a significant decrease in fracture risk was observed with use of metformin and sulphonylureas, and a non-significant trend towards decreased risk of any fracture when insulin was prescribed.

In "The Health, Aging, and Body Composition Study", Strotmeyer et al. concluded that T2D had a higher fracture risk (RR = 1.64) after adjustment for BMD and fracture risk factors in older, well-functioning males and females [39]. Furthermore, the authors concluded that a higher incidence of impaired sensation and transient ischemia attack were noted in patients with T2D and fractures than those without fracture. However, patients with IFG did not show significant fracture risk.

According to the results from "The Women's Health Initiative Observational Study", Bonds et al. concluded that the RR of overall fracture in these female patients was 1.2 compared with that in non-diabetic controls after adjusting for other fracture risk factors [42]. Furthermore, the risk was higher in the black population and in patients with high baseline BMD. Janghorbani et al. conducted the "The Nurses' Health Study" to determine the potential risk factors of further hip fractures [54]. Age-adjusted RR of hip fractures in patients with T2D was 1.7 compared with that in non-diabetic controls. However, the higher risk persisted even after controlling for other confounding factors. Furthermore, patients with long-term T2D (diabetic duration >12 years) and insulin use posed a greater risk to the future development of hip fractures. A systemic review by Janghorbani et al. suggested that T2D was associated with an increased risk of hip fractures with RR of 2.8 in male and 2.1 in female patients with T2D [55]. The fracture risk at other sites was weak. Similar results were noted in a meta-analysis performed by Vestergaard et al., in which patients with T2D increased RR to 1.38 as comparing to non-diabetic controls [26].

Recently, Melton et al. conducted a study to examine the potential effects of increased risk of hip fractures in subjects of T2D [58]. A total of 700 subjects with diabetes were analyzed during a follow-up of 23,226 person-years. The overall fracture risk calculated by standardized incidence ratios (SIRs) was 1.3, but the risk for hip fractures increased only when the follow-up duration exceeded 10 years. The high fracture risk was associated with old age, previous fracture history, and corticosteroid therapy. Conversely, increased physical activity and BMD had a protective role on fracture risk. The frequency of fractures increased among patients on insulin, decreased among patients on biquanides, and remained unaltered among patients on sulfonylurea or thiazolidinedione. A study by Koh et al., the "Singapore Chinese Health Study," was a prospective cohort study involving 63,257 Chinese patients with a mean age of 51.8 years and follow-up period of 12 years [59]. The RR of hip fracture in patients with diabetes was 1.98 compared with that in non-diabetic controls after controlling for other risk factors. The study also showed that diabetes duration was linearly associated with an increased risk of hip fractures.

2.3. Risk Factors of Fracture in Diabetes Mellitus

Similar to non-diabetic controls, those with DM (either T1D or T2D) had many fracture risk factors that were divided into modifiable and non-modifiable classifications. The Caucasian population, female gender, age, and family or personal history of fracture were non-modifiable etiologies that carried a higher risk for future bone fractures. Modifiable factors that could be prevented included smoking, excessive alcohol consumption, lean body mass, low calcium intake, hormone deficiency (estrogen or androgen), physical inactivity, chronic diseases, and medications. Diabetes was not included in the traditional fracture risk factors recommended by the WHO fracture risk assessment tool, FRAX [60]. Giangregorio et al. found that diabetes increased fracture risk independent of FRAX assessment of BMD, since patients with diabetes have an increased fracture risk due to other characteristics predisposing factors [61]. These included the presence of diabetic microangiopathy (including peripheral neuropathy and visual actuality impairment), hypoglycemia, nocturia, and dizziness due to medications. Although obesity plays a protective role in increasing BMD, high body size may counterbalance this protective effect. As mentioned previously, diabetes duration and use of anti-diabetic drugs (including insulin) were also associated with a higher fracture risk.

3. Association Mechanisms between DM and Osteoporosis

Several hypotheses have been proposed to explain the discrepancies in BMD in different types of diabetes. As previously mentioned, BMD is normal or increased in T2D and decreased in T1D. The exact mechanisms responsible for osteoporosis and fractures in both types of diabetes are not well known. Two major factors for maintaining bone structure are bone strength and bone quality. Bone remodeling involves a complex interaction between osteoblast and osteoclast function to maintain calcium balance for bone strength. It is generally accepted that chronic hyperglycemia, a major characteristic of both types of diabetes, and its consequences may interfere with the balance between osteoclast and osteoblast function.

3.1. Diabetic Complications

Many studies have determined that diabetic complications are associated with decreased BMD in patients with T1D [17,22-24]. Therefore, there had been hypothesized that diabetic microangiopahty [62] and macroangiopathy [63] link with the low BMD in T1D patients. Campos et al. observed that the presence of diabetic retinopathy may play an important role in the development of diabetic osteopenia [17]. Clausen et al. measured BMD in male patients with T1D at different stages of albuminuria, and the results suggested that microalbuminuria was an early indicator of diabetic osteopenia [64]. Rix et al. evaluated the influence of diabetic neuropathy on BMD in male patients with T1D and suggested that the severity of neuropathy was an independent risk factor for decreased BMD [65]. Similarly, the presence of peripheral vascular disorders also suggested that patients with T1D had decreased BMD [22]. Increased bone resorption may be a possible mechanism responsible for decreased BMD in patients with T1D. Levels of urinary hydroxyproline, a marker of bone resorption, in patients with T1D and microalbuminuria are higher than those in subjects with T1D and without microalbuminuria [66]. Furthermore, chronic complications resulted from chronic hyperglycemia and inadequate glycemic control resulted in increased bone resorption, meanwhile improved metabolic control should decrease bone resorption [14,17].

3.2. Insulin and Insulin-like Growth Factor-1

Insulin is a candidate factor to explain the decreased BMD in T1D since studies have reported that BMD in patients with T1D is lower than that in patients with T2D [13,18]. Tuominen et al. concluded that decreased BMD was probably due to accelerated bone loss after T1D onset [18]. Decreased BMD in patients with T1D suggested that insulin may play a role in bone metabolism. However, direct evidence of this association is weak. An animal study revealed that insulin receptor substrate-1 (IRS-1) deficiency impaired bone healing by inhibiting chondrocyte proliferation [67]. IRS-1 is essential for intracellular signaling by insulin and insulin-like growth factor-1 (IGF-1). Ogata et al. found that IRS-1 was expressed in osteoblasts, but not in osteoclasts, in wild-type mice. IRS-1 deficiency impaired osteoblast proliferation, differentiation, and osteoclastogenesis, which resulted in low bone turnover and osteopenia [68]. A recent study showed that spontaneous IRS-1 mutations in mice could induce impaired adipogenesis and low bone mass [69]. Dixit et al. reported that bone strength in patients with diabetes was lower than that in non-diabetic controls, but bone cortical thickness improved after insulin therapy, which suggested that insulin may offer some beneficial effects to bony structures [70]. These findings may suggest that insulin is an anabolic agent and important for bone metabolism [71].

IGF-1, a hormone with a similar molecular structure to insulin, plays a vital role in growth during childhood and continues to have anabolic effects in adulthood [72]. Several studies have found that serum IGF-1 or insulin growth factor-binding protein-3 (IGFBP-3) levels in patients with T1D were lower than those in patients with T2D or non-diabetic controls [20,73]. These markers are also positively associated with BMD [73]; however, a second study found that decreased BMD was not positively associated with bone markers, including IGF-1 and IGFBP-3, in patients with DM [16].

Nevertheless, osteoblasts have insulin and IGF-1 receptors [74]. Perrini et al. examined the action of IGF-1 in bone cells and its involvement in osteoporosis. They concluded that in patients with osteoporosis, impaired osteoblast proliferation may have resulted from dysregulation of IGF-I receptor signaling through several insulin signal pathways [75].

3.3. Peroxisome Proliferator-Activated Receptor Gamma

The decrease in BMD is mainly age-related in primary osteoporosis, which is often accompanied by an increase in bone marrow adipose tissue [76]. Several studies have suggested that osteoclastogenesis and adipogenesis share similar pathways [77,78]. Peroxisome proliferator-activated receptor gamma (PPAR-γ) is a transcription factor involved in adipocyte differentiation. In PPAR-γ heterozygous-deficient mice, trabecular bone volume increased, but bone marrow fat decreased, thus illustrating a protective mechanism for preventing bone loss through the stimulation of osteoblastogenesis [79]. Thiazolidinediones (TZDs) are oral anti-diabetic agents that act as insulin sensitizers via the activation of PPAR-γ. Rosiglitazone (ROS) is a TZD for management of hyperglycemia in subjects with T2D. Treatment with ROS in mice caused bone loss by suppressing osteoblast differentiation and bone formation [80]. This negative regulator effect on bone mass is an important mechanism to explain age-related osteoporosis. This concept was confirmed by another study [81]. A study using a streptozotocin-induced diabetic mouse model found that decreased bone mass occurred through changes in bone marrow composition resulting in decreased mature osteoblasts and increased adipose accumulation [82]. Similar results were reported in animal models with decreasing BMD that were treated with ROS [83,84].

Results of previous studies on fracture risk due to TZD therapy were inconsistent. Melton et al. noted that TZD therapy did not carry an increased fracture risk, but metformin therapy decreased fracture risk [58]. A cohort study involving a large elderly population (age, 70–79 years) suggested that TZD therapy for more than 24 months may decrease BMD [85]. Bone loss and/or bone fracture in patients with T2D during TZD treatment was not fully investigated until the prospective study called "A Diabetes Outcome Progression Trial" (ADOPT). In this study, patients treated with ROS had a higher fracture risk than those treated with glyburide or metformin [86]. TZD-related changes in bone markers were shown in short-term ROS therapy in postmenopausal female patients with diabetes and non-diabetic controls [87, 88]. The ADPOT study also analyzed changes in bone markers during drug therapies and found that changes in bone resorption markers may be partly responsible for the increased fracture risk in females treated with ROS [89]. TZDs may also affect bone metabolism by decreasing the circulating levels of IGF-1 and estrogen [90]. The latest meta-analysis confirmed that TZD-related bone loss or fracture risk may be a class effect, which can be noted in other types of TZDs (i.e., pioglitazone) [90].

3.4. Osteoprotegerin

Osteoprotegerin (OPG) and its ligand, known as receptor activator of NF-kappaB ligand (RANKL), are adipocytokines that serve as regulators of osteoclast function, including differentiation, activity, and survival [92-94]. Interaction between OPG and RANKL plays a vital role in bone remodeling in healthy individuals and those with certain diseases, including diabetes [95]. The association between serum OPG levels and BMD was inconclusive according to previous studies. Some studies showed that OPG levels were negatively associated with BMD in postmenopausal females [96], whereas they were positively associated in the elderly [97]. Furthermore, other studies did not find any association between OPG levels and BMD [98,99]. These conflicting results were also observed in patients with diabetes. OPG levels were increased in children with T1D [100,101], and its levels were found to be negatively associated with bone quality [101]. However, OPG levels in patients with T1D with normoalbuminuria were lower than those in non-diabetic controls [102]. This was similar to that in patients with T2D, where serum OPG levels were not positively associated with BMD and vertebral fractures [103]. Therefore, it is difficult to draw a accurate conclusion on the effect of OPG levels on BMD in diabetes. Some have suggested that it may be merely a marker for decreasing bone quality.

3.5. Advanced Glycation end Products and their Receptors

Production of advanced glycation end products (AGEs) in collagen results from chronic hyperglycemia, which is associated with the development of chronic vascular complications in diabetes [104]. Increasing evidence suggest that AGEs and their receptors (RAGEs) have detrimental effects on vascular wall via the generation of oxidative stress. AGE accumulation also influences osteoblasts and osteoclasts via inflammatory responses and has negative effects on bone metabolism by inhibiting synthesis of type-1 collagen and altering osteoblasts and osteoclast function, which includes inhibiting differentiation and mineralization in osteoblasts and enhancing osteoclast activity [105,106]. AGE accumulation in diabetes may accelerate apoptosis of osteoblasts, thereby resulting in diminished bone formation [107]. Furthermore, higher levels of AGE levels in collagen may alter bone strength and quality. Saito suggested that collagen cross-links serve as determinants of bone quality [108]. Pentosidine is a biomarker for AGEs and its contents in bone negatively associated with poor mechanical properties in some studies [109,110]. Pentosidine content of cortical and trabecular bone derived from patients with bone fractures was higher than that in normal controls [111]. Recent studies revealed that circulating pentosidine levels were positively associated with fracture risk in diabetes [112,113]. Interaction between AGEs and RAGE can induce oxidative stress resulting in decreased BMD. A recent study showed that low serum endogenous secretory RAGE levels was a risk factor for vertebral fractures independent of BMD in patients with T2D [114].

4. Evaluation and Treatment of Osteoporosis in Diabetes Mellitus

There are no formal guidelines or recommendations describing the evaluation and treatment of osteoporosis in DM. However, procedures should be similar to treatments of those without diabetes.

4.1. Risk Factor Detection, Evaluation, and Prevention

The National Osteoporosis Foundation (NOF) recommends that all postmenopausal females and males over the age of 50 should undergo osteoporosis risk assessments [115]. Subjects of T1D and T2D are associated with fracture risk, although BMD in T2D is higher than that in T1D. Therefore, patients with diabetes should be evaluated in the same manner as the general population. Furthermore, it may be necessary for early detection of osteoporosis, especially in patients with T1D. There are several conditions, diseases, and medications that may cause or contribute to osteoporosis, and fractures should be evaluated for osteoporosis and DM. However, it may not be feasible to evaluate patients with diabetes for osteoporosis and/or fracture risk using these criteria.

The hip fracture risk prediction tool FRAX proposed by the WHO did not consider diabetes as a risk factor [116]. Giangregorio et al. examined whether diabetes was a risk factor for incident hip or major osteoporotic fractures independent of FRAX assessment. Subjects with diabetes (n = 3518) and those without diabetes (n = 36,085) over 50 years were enrolled in the study [61]. The study confirmed that diabetes confers an increased fracture risk that is independent of FRAX assessment and suggested that the fracture risk in diabetes may be underestimated. The QFractureScore algorithm, which is used to estimate the risk of developing a hip fracture, included T2D as a significant factor, and it predicted an increase of 38% to 67% in fracture risk in patients with diabetic men and women as comparing to non-diabetic controls [117]. The clinical manifestations of osteoporosis are often silent before the occurrence of a fracture. One in 5 females is not diagnosed with osteoporosis despite presenting with a fracture. The presence of a previous fracture between the ages of 20 and 50 years is associated with a 74% increase in future fracture risk after the age of 50 years in the general population [118]. This risk should be higher in patients with DM. Other than the fracture risk factors in the general population, patients with diabetes have several other risk factors precipitating a fracture, which include impaired visual ability, deteriorated polyneuropathy, and nocturia. According to the recommendation of clinical guidelines, DEXA measurement is the best tool for screening and diagnosis of osteoporosis. However, it is not a perfect diagnostic tool because bone quality and geometry cannot be evaluated by DEXA, which is particularly true in patients with T2D because they have increased BMD. Therefore, comprehensive risk assessment for osteoporosis should go beyond BMD measurements. This is particularly true when assessing patients with diabetes.

All subjects with diabetes should be evaluated for primary and secondary osteoporosis when presenting with low trauma fractures. Primary osteoporosis is often age-related and frequently occurs in postmenopausal females and the elderly. Several medical conditions, diseases, and medications can cause secondary osteoporosis, which is also true for patients with T2D, who may have several endocrine disorders such as clinical manifestations of glucose intolerance (e.g., Cushing's syndrome, thyroid disorders, and adrenal disorders). All patients should have a detailed history taken and physical examination with a focus on the potential etiology of secondary osteoporosis.

4.2. Treatment and Prevention of Osteoporosis in Diabetes

Strategies used to treat osteoporosis in patients with diabetes are similar to those used to treat non-diabetic controls, which include non-pharmacological and pharmacological interventions.

4.2.1. Non-pharmacological Intervention

Non-pharmacological management of osteoporosis includes nutrition supplementation, exercise, and lifestyle modifications. Diet and nutritional supplementation of calcium and vitamin D is important to maintain bone quality. Notably, vitamin D plays a vital role in calcium absorption. The recommended amount of calcium and vitamin supplementation varies with gender, age, and pregnancy status. Regular exercise, particularly weight-bearing exercise, is beneficial for bone mass and to prevent bone loss and the risk of falling. Exercise offers additional beneficial effects especially in patients with T2D such as improved glycemic control via improvement of insulin sensitivity. Furthermore, adopting a healthy lifestyle is important for prevention and treatment of osteoporosis. Smoking and excessive alcohol consumption are well-documented risk factors for osteoporosis development. A healthy lifestyle is also helpful in management of diabetes and identifying risk factors for both osteoporosis and fracture risk, and are paramount for patients with T2D.

4.2.2. Pharmacological Intervention

Although patients with T1D and T2D have high osteoporotic and fracture risks, routine initiation of preventive medication is not recommended based on current evidence. According to the NOF guide, physicians should consider pharmacotherapy in postmenopausal females and males aged 50 years and older, based on the following: (1) a hip or vertebral (clinical or morphometric) fracture; (2) a T-score ≤ -2.5 at the femoral neck or spine after appropriate evaluation to exclude secondary causes; (3) low bone mass (T-score between -1.0 and -2.5 at the femoral neck or spine) and a 10-year probability of a hip fracture $\geq 3\%$ or a 10-year probability of a major osteoporosis-related fracture $\geq 20\%$ based on the US-adapted WHO algorithm [115]. This also holds true for subjects with diabetes. However, evidence-based pharmacotherapy recommendations for osteoporosis in subjects with diabetes are not available.

Several types of pharmacologic options have been approved by the Food and Drug Administration (FDA) for the prevention and/or treatment of osteoporosis, including estrogen, bisphosphonates, calcitonin, selective estrogen modulator (SERM) (i.e., raloxifene), and parathyroid hormone (PTH) (1-34). Estrogen, the major component of hormone replacement therapy, has been considered as the treatment of choice for osteoporosis because it improves BMD [119]. However, the indication of estrogen treatment for osteoporosis has been removed by the FDA due to a lack of fracture risk reduction in clinical trials. Other approved medications are available for management of osteoporosis, especially postmenopausal osteoporosis. Raloxifene is indicated for treatment and prevention of osteoporosis. It has organ-specific effects that differ from estrogen to minimize the side effects and cancer risk. Salmon calcitonin is a synthetic polypeptide and its effects are more potent than human calcitonin on bone osteoclasts via inhibition of osteoclast-induced bone resorption. Bisphosphonates are used most often worldwide for treatment and prevention of osteoporosis and bone fracture through inhibition of osteoclast function and decreasing bone turnover. PTH is a potent anabolic agent for management of osteoporosis by intermittent PTH injection. It should be considered that these drugs are used for osteoporosis; however, some possible effects on diabetes may occur. Most of these medications did not influence glycemic control, except for calcitonin, which was reported to have a hyperglycemic effect via inhibition of insulin secretion [120]. One report showed that alendronate, a biphosphonate, may decrease daily insulin requirements among patients with DM and osteoporosis in a small clinical trial [121]. Finally, a few novel medications have focused on inhibiting excessive bone resorption and increasing bone formation, including a monoclonal antibody for the receptor activator of the NF-κB ligand, a key osteoclast cytokine; odanacatib, a specific inhibitor of the osteoclast protease cathepsin K; and antibodies against the proteins sclerostin and dickkopf-1, 2 endogenous inhibitors of bone formation that have been recognized in management of osteoporosis [122]. Again, the specific role of osteoporosis in patients with diabetes is lacking. Patients with low-impact fractures or osteoporosis should be offered treatment including non-pharmacological and pharmacological therapies. Many agents are available for the prevention and treatment of osteoporosis in the diabetic population. The decision to initiate therapy should be individualized.

CONCLUSION

Both DM and osteoporosis are highly prevalent diseases and also result in severe co-morbidity. Both diseases are clinically silent during the early stage of the natural disease course. At present, osteoporosis is considered a complication of DM, and conversely, DM is a significant risk factor for the development of osteoporosis. Therefore, it is necessary to identify high-risk patients and prevent and aggressively treat both diseases simultaneously. BMD measurement by DEXA in diabetes is not feasible as using in the general population. Physicians should be aware of diabetes-related risk factors or markers of osteoporosis. Currently, there are no available specific guidelines or recommendations for the management of osteoporosis in patients with diabetes; hence, the management strategy for osteoporosis and bone fractures is the same as in non-diabetic controls. Further clinical evidence concerning screening and management of osteoporosis in patients with diabetes is needed.

REFERENCES

[1] Assessment of fracture risk and its application to screening for postmenopausal osteoporosis. Report of a WHO Study Group. *World Health Organ Tech Rep Ser* 1994;843: 1-129.

[2] Rosen CJ. Endocrine disorders and osteoporosis. *Curr Opin Rheumatol* 1997;9: 355-61.

[3] Kanis JA, Melton LJ 3rd, Christiansen C, Johnston CC, Khaltaev N. The diagnosis of osteoporosis. *J Bone Miner Res* 1994;9: 1137-41.

[4] Gunczler P, Lanes R, Paoli M, Martinis R, Villaroel O, Weisinger JR. Decreased bone mineral density and bone formation markers shortly after diagnosis of clinical type 1 diabetes mellitus. *J Pediatr Endocrinol Metab* 2001;14: 525-8.

[5] Gunczler P, Lanes R, Paz-Martinez V, Martins R, Esaa S, Colmenares V, Weisinger JR. Decreased lumbar spine bone mass and low bone turnover in children and adolescents with insulin dependent diabetes mellitus followed longitudinally. *J Pediatr Endocrinol Metab* 1998;11: 413-9.

[6] Ersoy B, Gökşen D, Darcan S, Mavi E, Oztürk C. Evaluation of bone mineral density in children with diabetes mellitus. *Indian J Pediatr* 1999;66: 375-9.

[7] Lettgen B, Hauffa B, Mohlmann C, Jeken C, Reiners C. Bone mineral density in children and adolescents with juvenile diabetes: selective measurement of bone mineral density of trabecular and cortical bone using peripheral quantitative computed tomography. *Horm Res* 1995;43: 173-5.
[8] Heap J, Murray MA, Miller SC, Jalili T, Moyer-Mileur LJ. Alterations in bone characteristics associated with glycemic control in adolescents with type 1 diabetes mellitus. *J Pediatr* 2004;144: 56-62.
[9] Liu EY, Wactawski-Wende J, Donahue RP, Dmochowski J, Hovey KM, Quattrin T. Does low bone mineral density start in post-teenage years in women with type 1 diabetes? *Diabetes Care* 2003;26: 2365-9.
[10] Valerio G, del Puente A, Esposito-del Puente A, Buono P, Mozzillo E, Franzese A. The lumbar bone mineral density is affected by long-term poor metabolic control in adolescents with type 1 diabetes mellitus. *Horm Res* 2002;58: 266-72.
[11] Heilman K, Zilmer M, Zilmer K, Tillmann V. Lower bone mineral density in children with type 1 diabetes is associated with poor glycemic control and higher serum ICAM-1 and urinary isoprostane levels. *J Bone Miner Metab* 2009;27: 598-604.
[12] Saha MT, Sievänen H, Salo MK, Tulokas S, Saha HH. Bone mass and structure in adolescents with type 1 diabetes compared to healthy peers. *Osteoporos Int* 2009;20: 1401-6.
[13] Christensen JO, Svendsen OL. Bone mineral in pre- and postmenopausal women with insulin-dependent and non-insulin-dependent diabetes mellitus. *Osteoporos Int* 1999;10: 307-11.
[14] Krakauer JC, McKenna MJ, Buderer NF, Rao DS, Whitehouse FW, Parfitt AM. Bone loss and bone turnover in diabetes. *Diabetes* 1995;44: 75-82.
[15] Miazgowski T, Czekalski S. A 2-year follow-up study on bone mineral density and markers of bone turnover in patients with long-standing insulin-dependent diabetes mellitus. *Osteoporos Int* 1998;8: 399-403.
[16] Mastrandrea LD, Wactawski-Wende J, Donahue RP, Hovey KM, Clark A, Quattrin T. Young women with type 1 diabetes have lower bone mineral density that persists over time. *Diabetes Care* 2008;31: 1729-35.
[17] Campos Pastor MM, López-Ibarra PJ, Escobar-Jiménez F, Serrano Pardo MD, García-Cervigón AG. Intensive insulin therapy and bone mineral density in type 1 diabetes mellitus: a prospective study. *Osteoporos Int* 2000;11: 455-9.

[18] Tuominen JT, Impivaara O, Puukka P, Rönnemaa T. Bone mineral density in patients with type 1 and type 2 diabetes. *Diabetes Care* 1999;22: 1196-200.

[19] López-Ibarra PJ, Pastor MM, Escobar-Jiménez F, Pardo MD, González AG, Luna JD, Requena ME, Diosdado MA. Bone mineral density at time of clinical diagnosis of adult-onset type 1 diabetes mellitus. *Endocr Pract* 2001;7: 346-51.

[20] Kemink SA, Hermus AR, Swinkels LM, Lutterman JA, Smals AG. Osteopenia in insulin-dependent diabetes mellitus; prevalence and aspects of pathophysiology. *J Endocrinol Invest* 2000;23: 295-303.

[21] Kayath MJ, Tavares EF, Dib SA, Vieira JG. Prospective bone mineral density evaluation in patients with insulin-dependent diabetes mellitus. *J Diabetes Complications* 1998;12: 133-9.

[22] Muñoz-Torres M, Jódar E, Escobar-Jiménez F, López-Ibarra PJ, Luna JD. Bone mineral density measured by dual X-ray absorptiometry in Spanish patients with insulin-dependent diabetes mellitus. *Calcif Tissue Int* 1996;58: 316-9.

[23] Rozadilla A, Nolla JM, Montaña E, Fiter J, Gómez-Vaquero C, Soler J, Roig-Escofet D. Bone mineral density in patients with type 1 diabetes mellitus. *Joint Bone Spine* 2000;67: 215-8.

[24] Lunt H, Florkowski CM, Cundy T, Kendall D, Brown LJ, Elliot JR, Wells JE, Turner JG. A population-based study of bone mineral density in women with longstanding type 1 (insulin dependent) diabetes. *Diabetes Res Clin Pract* 1998;40: 31-8.

[25] Hamilton EJ, Rakic V, Davis WA, Chubb SA, Kamber N, Prince RL, Davis TM. Prevalence and predictors of osteopenia and osteoporosis in adults with Type 1 diabetes. *Diabet Med* 2009;26: 45-52.

[26] Vestergaard P. Discrepancies in bone mineral density and fracture risk in patients with type 1 and type 2 diabetes-a meta-analysis. *Osteoporos Int* 2007;18: 427–44.

[27] Hadjidakis DJ, Raptis AE, Sfakianakis M, Mylonakis A, Raptis SA. Bone mineral density of both genders in Type 1 diabetes according to bone composition. *J Diabetes Complications* 2006;20: 302-7.

[28] Bridges MJ, Moochhala SH, Barbour J, Kelly CA. Influence of diabetes on peripheral bone mineral density in men: a controlled study. *Acta Diabetol* 2005;42: 82-6.

[29] Räkel A, Sheehy O, Rahme E, LeLorier J. Osteoporosis among patients with type 1 and type 2 diabetes. *Diabetes Metab* 2008;34: 193-205.

[30] van Daele PL, Stolk RP, Burger H, Algra D, Grobbee DE, Hofman A, Birkenhäger JC, Pols HA. Bone density in non-insulin-dependent diabetes mellitus. The Rotterdam Study. *Ann Intern Med* 1995;122: 409-14.

[31] Barrett-Connor E, Holbrook TL. Sex differences in osteoporosis in older adults with non-insulin-dependent diabetes mellitus. *JAMA* 1992;268: 3333-7.

[32] Rishaug U, Birkeland KI, Falch JA, Vaaler S. Bone mass in non-insulin-dependent diabetes mellitus. *Scand J Clin Lab Invest* 1995;55: 257-62.

[33] Kwon DJ, Kim JH, Chung KW, Kim JH, Lee JW, Kim SP, Lee HY.Bone mineral density of the spine using dual energy X-ray absorptiometry in patients with non-insulin-dependent diabetes mellitus. *J Obstet Gynaecol Res* 1996;22: 157-62.

[34] el Miedany YM, el Gaafary S, el Baddini MA. Osteoporosis in older adults with non-insulin-dependent diabetes mellitus: is it sex related? *Clin Exp Rheumatol* 1999;17: 561-7.

[35] Isaia GC, Ardissone P, Di Stefano M, Ferrari D, Martina V, Porta M, Tagliabue M, Molinatti GM. Bone metabolism in type 2 diabetes mellitus. *Acta Diabetol* 1999;36: 35-8.

[36] Schwartz AV, Sellmeyer DE, Ensrud KE, Cauley JA, Tabor HK, Schreiner PJ, Jamal SA, Black DM, Cummings SR; Study of Osteoporotic Features Research Group. Older women with diabetes have an increased risk of fracture: a prospective study. *J Clin Endocrinol Metab* 2001;86: 32-8.

[37] Sert M, Tetiker T, Kirim S, Soyupak S, Canataroğlu A, Koçak M. Type 2 diabetes mellitus and osteopenia: is there an association? *Acta Diabetol* 2003;40: 105-8.

[38] Kao WH, Kammerer CM, Schneider JL, Bauer RL, Mitchell BD. Type 2 diabetes is associated with increased bone mineral density in Mexican-American women. *Arch Med Res* 2003;34: 399-406.

[39] Strotmeyer ES, Cauley JA, Schwartz AV, Nevitt MC, Resnick HE, Zmuda JM, Bauer DC, Tylavsky FA, de Rekeneire N, Harris TB, Newman AB; Health ABC Study. Diabetes is associated independently of body composition with BMD and bone volume in older white and black men and women: The Health, Aging, and Body Composition Study. *J Bone Miner Res* 2004;19: 1084-91.

[40] Dennison EM, Syddall HE, Aihie Sayer A, Craighead S, Phillips DI, Cooper C. Type 2 diabetes mellitus is associated with increased axial bone density in men and women from the Hertfordshire Cohort Study:

evidence for an indirect effect of insulin resistance? *Diabetologia* 2004;47: 1963-8.

[41] de Liefde II, van der Klift M, de Laet CE, van Daele PL, Hofman A, Pols HA. Bone mineral density and fracture risk in type-2 diabetes mellitus: the Rotterdam Study. *Osteoporos Int* 2005;16: 1713-20.

[42] Bonds DE, Larson JC, Schwartz AV, Strotmeyer ES, Robbins J, Rodriguez BL, Johnson KC, Margolis KL. Risk of fracture in women with type 2 diabetes: the Women's Health Initiative Observational Study. *J Clin Endocrinol Metab* 2006;91: 3404-10.

[43] Khalil N, Sutton-Tyrrell K, Strotmeyer ES, Greendale GA, Vuga M, Selzer F, Crandall CJ, Cauley JA. Menopausal bone changes and incident fractures in diabetic women: a cohort study. *Osteoporos Int* 2011;22: 1367-76.

[44] Schwartz AV, Vittinghoff E, Bauer DC, Hillier TA, Strotmeyer ES, Ensrud KE, Donaldson MG, Cauley JA, Harris TB, Koster A, Womack CR, Palermo L, Black DM; Study of Osteoporotic Fractures (SOF) Research Group; Osteoporotic Fractures in Men (MrOS) Research Group; Health, Aging, and Body Composition (Health ABC) Research Group. Association of BMD and FRAX score with risk of fracture in older adults with type 2 diabetes. *JAMA* 2011;305: 2184-92.

[45] Sosa M, Dominguez M, Navarro MC, Segarra MC, Hernández D, de Pablos P, Betancor P. Bone mineral metabolism is normal in non-insulin-dependent diabetes mellitus. *J Diabetes Complications* 1996;10: 201-5.

[46] Hampson G, Evans C, Petitt RJ, Evans WD, Woodhead SJ, Peters JR, Ralston SH. Bone mineral density, collagen type 1 alpha 1 genotypes and bone turnover in premenopausal women with diabetes mellitus. *Diabetologia* 1998;41: 1314-20.

[47] Majima T, Komatsu Y, Yamada T, Koike Y, Shigemoto M, Takagi C, Hatanaka I, Nakao K. Decreased bone mineral density at the distal radius, but not at the lumbar spine or the femoral neck, in Japanese type 2 diabetic patients. *Osteoporos Int* 2005;16: 907-13.

[48] Al-Maatouq MA, El-Desouki MI, Othman SA, Mattar EH, Babay ZA, Addar M. Prevalence of osteoporosis among postmenopausal females with diabetes mellitus. *Saudi Med J* 2004;25: 1423-7.

[49] Lee JH, Lee YH, Jung KH, Kim MK, Jang HW, Kim TK, Kim HJ, Jo YS, Shong M, Lee TY, Ku BJ. Bone mineral density in prediabetic men. *Korean Diabetes J* 2010;34: 294-302.

[50] Forsén L, Meyer HE, Midthjell K, Edna TH. Diabetes mellitus and the incidence of hip fracture: results from the Nord-Trøndelag Health Survey. *Diabetologia* 1999;42: 920-5.

[51] Nicodemus KK, Folsom AR; Iowa Women's Health Study. Type 1 and type 2 diabetes and incident hip fractures in postmenopausal women. *Diabetes Care* 2001;24: 1192-7.

[52] Miao J, Brismar K, Nyrén O, Ugarph-Morawski A, Ye W. Elevated hip fracture risk in type 1 diabetic patients: a population-based cohort study in Sweden. *Diabetes Care* 2005;28: 2850-5.

[53] Vestergaard P, Rejnmark L, Mosekilde L. Relative fracture risk in patients with diabetes mellitus, and the impact of insulin and oral antidiabetic medication on relative fracture risk. *Diabetologia* 2005;48: 1292-9.

[54] Janghorbani M, Feskanich D, Willett WC, Hu F. Prospective study of diabetes and risk of hip fracture: the Nurses' Health Study. *Diabetes Care* 2006;29: 1573-8.

[55] Janghorbani M, Van Dam RM, Willett WC, Hu FB. Systematic review of type 1 and type 2 diabetes mellitus and risk of fracture. *Am J Epidemiol* 2007;166: 495-505.

[56] Ivers RQ, Cumming RG, Mitchell P, Peduto AJ; Blue Mountains Eye Study. Diabetes and risk of fracture: The Blue Mountains Eye Study. *Diabetes Care* 2001;24: 1198-203.

[57] Ottenbacher KJ, Ostir GV, Peek MK, Goodwin JS, Markides KS. Diabetes mellitus as a risk factor for hip fracture in mexican american older adults. *J Gerontol A Biol Sci Med Sci* 2002;57: M648-53.

[58] Melton LJ 3rd, Leibson CL, Achenbach SJ, Therneau TM, Khosla S. Fracture risk in type 2 diabetes: update of a population-based study. *J Bone Miner Res* 2008;23: 1334-42.

[59] Koh WP, Wang R, Ang LW, Heng D, Yuan JM, Yu MC.Diabetes and risk of hip fracture in the Singapore Chinese Health Study. *Diabetes Care* 2010;33: 1766-70.

[60] Http://www.shef.ac.uk/FRAX/

[61] Giangregorio LM, Leslie WD, Lix LM, Johansson H, Oden A, McCloskey E, Kanis JA. FRAX underestimates fracture risk in patients with diabetes. *J Bone Miner Res* 2012;27: 301-8.

[62] Yamagishi S, Nakamura K, Inoue H. Possible participation of advanced glycation end products in the pathogenesis of osteoporosis in diabetic patients. *Med Hypotheses* 2005;65: 1013-5.

[63] Vogt MT, Cauley JA, Kuller LH, Nevitt MC. Bone mineral density and blood flow to the lower extremities: the study of osteoporotic fractures. *J Bone Miner Res* 1997;12: 283-9.

[64] Clausen P, Feldt-Rasmussen B, Jacobsen P, Rossing K, Parving HH, Nielsen PK, Feldt-Rasmussen U, Olgaard K. Microalbuminuria as an early indicator of osteopenia in male insulin-dependent diabetic patients. *Diabet Med* 1997;14: 1038-43.

[65] Rix M, Andreassen H, Eskildsen P. Impact of peripheral neuropathy on bone density in patients with type 1 diabetes. *Diabetes Care* 1999;22: 827-31

[66] Selby PL, Shearing PA, Marshall SM. Hydroxyproline excretion is increased in diabetes mellitus and related to the presence of microalbuminuria. *Diabet Med* 1995;12: 240-3.

[67] Shimoaka T, Kamekura S, Chikuda H, Hoshi K, Chung UI, Akune T, Maruyama Z, Komori T, Matsumoto M, Ogawa W, Terauchi Y, Kadowaki T, Nakamura K, Kawaguchi H. Impairment of bone healing by insulin receptor substrate-1 deficiency. *J Biol Chem* 2004;279: 15314-22.

[68] Ogata N, Chikazu D, Kubota N, Terauchi Y, Tobe K, Azuma Y, Ohta T, Kadowaki T, Nakamura K, Kawaguchi H. Insulin receptor substrate-1 in osteoblast is indispensable for maintaining bone turnover. *J Clin Invest* 2000;105: 935-43.

[69] DeMambro VE, Kawai M, Clemens TL, Fulzele K, Maynard JA, Marín de Evsikova C, Johnson KR, Canalis E, Beamer WG, Rosen CJ, Donahue LR. A novel spontaneous mutation of Irs1 in mice results in hyperinsulinemia, reduced growth, low bone mass and impaired adipogenesis. *J Endocrinol* 2010;204: 241-53.

[70] Dixit PK, Ekstrom RA. Decreased breaking strength of diabetic rat bone and its improvement by insulin treatment. *Calcif Tissue Int* 1980;32: 195-9.

[71] Thrailkill KM, Lumpkin CK Jr, Bunn RC, Kemp SF, Fowlkes JL. Is insulin an anabolic agent in bone? Dissecting the diabetic bone for clues. *Am J Physiol Endocrinol Metab* 2005;289: E735-45.

[72] Thrailkill KM, Liu L, Wahl EC, Bunn RC, Perrien DS, Cockrell GE, Skinner RA, Hogue WR, Carver AA, Fowlkes JL, Aronson J, Lumpkin CK Jr. Bone formation is impaired in a model of type 1 diabetes. *Diabetes* 2005;54: 2875-81.

[73] Jehle PM, Jehle DR, Mohan S, Böhm BO. Serum levels of insulin-like growth factor system components and relationship to bone metabolism

in Type 1 and Type 2 diabetes mellitus patients. *J Endocrinol* 1998;159: 297-306.

[74] Raisz LG. Local and systemic factors in the pathogenesis of osteoporosis. *N Engl J Med 1988*;318: 818–28.

[75] Perrini S, Natalicchio A, Laviola L, Cignarelli A, Melchiorre M, De Stefano F, Caccioppoli C, Leonardini A, Martemucci S, Belsanti G, Miccoli S, Ciampolillo A, Corrado A, Cantatore FP, Giorgino R, Giorgino F. Abnormalities of insulin-like growth factor-I signaling and impaired cell proliferation in osteoblasts from subjects with osteoporosis. *Endocrinology* 2008;149: 302-13.

[76] Rozman C, Feliu E, Berga L, Reverter JC, Climent C, Ferran MJ. Agerelated variations of fat tissue fraction in normal human bone marrow depend both on size and number of adipocytes: a stereological study. *Exp Hematol* 1989;17: 34–7.

[77] Gimble JM, Robinson CE, Wu X, Kelly KA. The function of adipocytes in the bone marrow stroma: an update. *Bone* 1996;19: 421-8.

[78] Nuttall ME, Gimble JM. Controlling the balance between osteoblastogenesis and adipogenesis and the consequent therapeutic implications. *Curr Opin Pharmacol* 2004; 4: 290-4.

[79] Akune T, Ohba S, Kamekura S, Yamaguchi M, Chung UI, Kubota N, Terauchi Y, Harada Y, Azuma Y, Nakamura K, Kadowaki T, Kawaguchi H. PPAR {gamma} insufficiency enhances osteogenesis through osteoblast formation from bone marrow progenitors. *J Clin Invest* 2004;113: 846-55.

[80] Ali AA, Weinstein RS, Stewart SA, Parfitt AM, Manolagas SC, Jilka RL. Rosiglitazone causes bone loss in mice by suppressing osteoblast differentiation and bone formation. *Endocrinology* 2005;146: 1226-35.

[81] Lazarenko OP, Rzonca SO, Hogue WR, Swain FL, Suva LJ, Lecka-Czernik B. Rosiglitazone induces decreases in bone mass and strength that are reminiscent of aged bone. *Endocrinology* 2007;148: 2669-80.

[82] Botolin S, Faugere MC, Malluche H, Orth M, Meyer R, McCabe LR. Increased bone adiposity and peroxisomal proliferator-activated receptor-gamma2 expression in type I diabetic mice. *Endocrinology* 2005;146: 3622-31.

[83] Soroceanu MA, Miao D, Bai XY, Su H, Goltzman D, Karaplis AC. Rosiglitazone impacts negatively on bone by promoting osteoblast/osteocyte apoptosis. *J Endocrinol* 2004;183: 203-16.

[84] Rzonca SO, Suva LJ, Gaddy D, Montague DC, Lecka-Czernik B. Bone is a target for the antidiabetic compound rosiglitazone. *Endocrinology* 2004;145: 401-6.

[85] Schwartz AV, Sellmeyer DE, Vittinghoff E, Palermo L, Lecka-Czernik B, Feingold KR, Strotmeyer ES, Resnick HE, Carbone L, Beamer BA, Park SW, Lane NE, Harris TB, Cummings SR. Thiazolidinedione use and bone loss in older diabetic adults. *J Clin Endocrinol Metab* 2006;91: 3349-54.

[86] Kahn SE, Haffner SM, Heise MA, Herman WH, Holman RR, Jones NP, Kravitz BG, Lachin JM, O'Neill MC, Zinman B, Viberti G; ADOPT Study Group. Glycemic durability of rosiglitazone, retformin, or glyburide monotherapy. *N Engl J Med* 2006;355: 2427-43.

[87] Berberoglu Z, Gursoy A, Bayraktar N, Yazici AC, Tutuncu NB, Demirag NG. Rosiglitazone decreases serum bone-specific alkaline phosphatase activity in postmenopausal diabetic women. *J Clin Endocrinol Metab* 2007;92: 3523-30.

[88] Grey A, Bolland M, Gamble G, Wattie D, Horne A, Davidson J, Reid IR. The peroxisome-proliferatoractivated receptor-gamma agonist rosiglitazone decreases bone formation and bone mineral density in healthy postmenopausal women: a randomized, controlled trial. *J Clin Endocrinol Metab* 2007;92: 1305-10.

[89] Zinman B, Haffner SM, Herman WH, Holman RR, Lachin JM, Kravitz BG, Paul G, Jones NP, Aftring RP, Viberti G, Kahn SE; ADOPT Study Group. Effect of rosiglitazone, metformin, and glyburide on bone biomarkers in patients with type 2 diabetes. *J Clin Endocrinol Metab* 2010;95: 134-42.

[90] Vestergaard P. Bone metabolism in type 2 diabetes and role of thiazolidinediones. *Curr Opin Endocrinol Diabetes Obes* 2009;16: 125-31.

[91] Meier C, Kraenzlin ME, Bodmer M, Jick SS, Jick H, Meier CR. Use of thiazolidinediones and fracture risk. *Arch Intern Med 2008*;168: 820-5.

[92] Simonet WS, Lacey DL, Dunstan CR, Kelley M, Chang MS, Lüthy R, Nguyen HQ, Wooden S, Bennett L, Boone T, Shimamoto G, DeRose M, Elliott R, Colombero A, Tan HL, Trail G, Sullivan J, Davy E, Bucay N, Renshaw-Gegg L, Hughes TM, Hill D, Pattison W, Campbell P, Sander S, Van G, Tarpley J, Derby P, Lee R, Boyle WJ. Osteoprotegerin: a novel secreted protein involved in the regulation of bone density. *Cell* 1997;89: 309-19.

[93] Lacey DL, Timms E, Tan HL, Kelley MJ, Dunstan CR, Burgess T, Elliott R, Colombero A, Elliott G, Scully S, Hsu H, Sullivan J, Hawkins N, Davy E, Capparelli C, Eli A, Qian YX, Kaufman S, Sarosi I, Shalhoub V, Senaldi G, Guo J, Delaney J, Boyle WJ. Osteoprotegerin ligand is a cytokine that regulates osteoclast differentiation and activation. *Cell* 1998;93: 165-76.
[94] Kong YY, Yoshida H, Sarosi I, Tan HL, Timms E, Capparelli C, Morony S, Oliveira-dos-Santos AJ, Van G, Itie A, Khoo W, Wakeham A, Dunstan CR, Lacey DL, Mak TW, Boyle WJ, Penninger JM. OPGL is a key regulator of osteoclastogenesis, lymphocyte development and lymph-node organogenesis. *Nature* 1999;397: 315-23.
[95] Kearns AE, Khosla S, Kostenuik PJ. Receptor activator of nuclear factor kappaB ligand and osteoprotegerin regulation of bone remodeling in health and disease. *Endocr Rev* 2008;29: 155-92.
[96] Jørgensen L, Vik A, Emaus N, Brox J, Hansen JB, Mathiesen E, Vestergaard P. Bone loss in relation to serum levels of osteoprotegerin and nuclear factor-kappaB ligand: the Tromso study. *Osteoporos Int* 2010;21: 931-8.
[97] Stern A, Laughlin GA, Bergstrom J, Barrett-Connor E. The sex-specific association of serum osteoprotegerin and receptor activator of nuclear factor kappaB legend with bone mineral density in older adults: the Rancho Bernardo study. *Eur J Endocrinol* 2007;156: 555-62.
[98] Indridason OS, Franzson L, Sigurdsson G. Serum osteoprotegerin and its relationship with bone mineral density and markers of bone turnover. *Osteoporos Int* 2005;16: 417-23.
[99] Liu JM, Zhao HY, Ning G, Zhao YJ, Chen Y, Zhang Zh, Sun LH, Xu MY, Chen JL. Relationships between the changes of serum levels of OPG and RANKL with age, menopause, bone biochemical markers and bone mineral density in Chinese women aged 20–75. *Calcif Tissue Int* 2005;76: 1-6.
[100] Alexopoulou O, Jamart J, Devogelaer JP, Brichard S, de Nayer P, Buysschaert M. Bone density and markers of bone remodeling in type 1 male diabetic patients. *Diabetes Metab* 2006;32: 453-8.
[101] Galluzzi F, Stagi S, Salti R, Toni S, Piscitelli E, Simonini G, Falcini F, Chiarelli F. Osteoprotegerin serum levels in children with type 1 diabetes: a potential modulating role in bone status. *Eur J Endocrinol* 2005;153: 879-85.

[102] Singh DK, Winocour P, Summerhayes B, Viljoen A, Sivakumar G, Farrington K. Low serum osteoprotegerin levels in normoalbuminuric type 1 diabetes mellitus. *Acta Diabetol* 2010;47(Suppl 1): 105-10.

[103] Rozas Moreno P, Reyes García R, García-Martín A, Varsavsky M, García-Salcedo JA, Muñoz-Torres M. Serum osteoprotegerin: bone or cardiovascular marker in type 2 diabetes males? *J Endocrinol Invest* 2012 Feb 28 [Epub ahead of print]

[104] Goldin A, Beckman JA, Schmidt AM, Creager MA. Advanced glycation end products sparking the development of diabetic vascular injury. *Circulation* 2006 114: 597-605.

[105] Katayama Y, Akatsu T, Yamamoto M, Kugai N, Nagata N. Role of nonenzymatic glycosylation of type 1 collagen in diabetic osteopenia. *J Bone Miner Res* 2006;11: 931-7.

[106] Sanguineti R, Storace D, Monacelli F, Federici A, Odetti P. Pentosidine effects on human osteoblasts in vitro. *Ann N Y Acad Sci* 2008;1126: 166-72.

[107] Alikhani M, Alikhani Z, Boyd C, MacLellan CM, Raptis M, Liu R, Pischon N, Trackman PC, Gerstenfeld L, Graves DT. Advanced glycation end products stimulate osteoblast apoptosis via the MAP kinase and cytosolic apoptotic pathways. *Bone* 2007;40: 345-53.

[108] Saito M, Marumo K. Collagen cross-links as a determinant of bone quality: a possible explanation for bone fragility in aging, osteoporosis, and diabetes mellitus. *Osteoporos Int* 2010;21: 195-214.

[109] Hernandez CJ, Tang SY, Baumbach BM, Hwu PB, Sakkee AN, van der Ham F, DeGroot J, Bank RA, Keaveny TM. Trabecular microfracture and the influence of pyridinium and non-enzymatic glycationmediated collagen cross-links. *Bone* 2005;37: 825-32.

[110] Viguet-Carrin S, Roux JP, Arlot ME, Merabet Z, Leeming DJ, Byrjalsen I, Delmas PD, Bouxsein ML. Contribution of the advanced glycation end product pentosidine and of maturation of type I collagen to compressive biomechanical properties of human lumbar vertebrae. *Bone* 2006;39: 1073-9.

[111] Saito M, Fujii K, Soshi S, Tanaka T. Reductions in degree of mineralization and enzymatic collagen cross-links and increases in glycation-induced pentosidine in the femoral neck cortex in cases of femoral neck fracture. *Osteoporos Int* 2006;17: 986-95.

[112] Yamamoto M, Yamaguchi T, Yamauchi M, Yano S, Sugimoto T. Serum pentosidine levels are positively associated with the presence of

vertebral fractures in postmenopausal women with type 2 diabetes. *J Clin Endocrinol Metab* 2008;93: 1013-9.

[113] Schwartz AV, Garnero P, Hillier TA, Sellmeyer DE, Strotmeyer ES, Feingold KR, Resnick HE, Tylavsky FA, Black DM, Cummings SR, Harris TB, Bauer DC; Health, Aging, and Body Composition Study. Pentosidine and increased fracture risk in older adults with type 2 diabetes. *J Clin Endocrinol Metab* 2009;94: 2380-6.

[114] Yamamoto M, Yamaguchi T, Yamauchi M, Sugimoto T. Low serum level of the endogenous secretory receptor for advanced glycation end products (esRAGE) is a risk factor for prevalent vertebral fractures independent of bone mineral density in patients with type 2 diabetes. *Diabetes Care* 2009;32: 2263-8.

[115] NOF Clinician's Guide to Prevention and Treatment of Osteoporosis. http://www.nof.org/professionals/clinical-guidelines.

[116] Kanis JA, Borgstrom F, De Laet C, Johansson H, Johnell O, Jonsson B, Oden A, Zethraeus N, Pfleger B, Khaltaev N. Assessment of fracture risk. *Osteoporos Int* 2005;16: 581-9.

[117] Hippisley-Cox J, Coupland C. Predicting risk of osteoporotic fracture in men and women in England and Wales: prospective derivation and validation of QFractureScores. *BMJ* 2009;339:b4229.

[118] Wu F, Mason B, Horne A, Ames R, Clearwater J, Liu M, Evans MC, Gamble GD, Reid IR: Fractures between the ages of 20 and 50 years increase women's risk of subsequent fractures. *Arch Intern Med* 2002;162: 33-6.

[119] Writing Group for the PEPI Trial: Effects of hormone therapy on bone mineral density: results from the Postmenopausal Estrogen/Progestin Interventions (PEPI) Trial. *JAMA* 1996; 276: 1389-96.

[120] Young AA, Wang MW, Gedulin B, Rink TJ, Pittner R, Beaumont K: Diabetogenic effects of salmon calcitonin are attributable to amylin-like activity. *Metabolism* 1995;44: 1581-9.

[121] Maugeri D, Panebianco P, Rosso D, Calanna A, Speciale S, Santangelo A, Rizza I, Motta M, Lentini A, Malaguarnera M: Alendronate reduces the daily consumption of insulin (DCI) in patients with senile type I diabetes and osteoporosis. *Arch Gerontol Geriatr* 2002;34: 117-22.

[122] Rachner TD, Khosla S, Hofbauer LC. Osteoporosis: now and the future. *Lancet* 2011;377: 1276-87.

In: Bone Loss
Editor: Kuo-Cheng Lu
ISBN: 978-1-62417-169-7

Chapter 3

BONE LOSS AND CARDIOVASCULAR DISEASE

***Jen-Yu Wang*[1] *and Kuo-Cheng Lu*[2]**

[1]Division of Cardiology, Department of Medicine, Cardinal Tien Hospital, School of Medicine, Fu Jen Catholic University, New Taipei City, Taiwan

[2]Division of Nephrology, Department of Medicine, Cardinal Tien Hospital, School of Medicine, Fu Jen Catholic University, New Taipei City, Taiwan

ABSTRACT

Traditionally, osteoporosis and cardiovascular disease (CVD) were thought to be separate chronic diseases. Accumulating evidence now supports a direct association between osteoporosis and hypertension, dyslipidemia, atherosclerosis, vascular calcification, and congestive heart failure. Significant advances have been made in recent years in elucidating the pathophysiological relationship and common risk factors between osteoporosis and CVD. An improved understanding of the pathophysiological mechanisms common to these conditions may contribute to future development of therapies that can act on both bone metabolism and CVD.

1. Introduction

Osteoporosis, a systemic skeletal disease characterized by decreased bone mineral density (BMD), can lead to bone fragility and increased susceptibility to fractures [1]. Because the prevalence rates of osteoporosis, atherosclerosis, hypertension, and cardiovascular (CV) disease (CVD) all increase with age, it is likely that these conditions will coexist more frequently in modern aging societies [2]. Traditionally, osteoporosis and CVD were thought to be separate chronic diseases. Both are major health problems resulting in significant morbidity and mortality. Accumulating evidence now supports a direct association between osteoporosis and CVD, independent of age or common CV risk factors [3-13].

Several retrospective analyses have shown significant associations between low BMD and atherosclerotic vascular disease independent of age, smoking, diabetes mellitus, or dyslipidemia [5, 6]. Results from a study by Sennerby et al. suggested a significant association between a receiving a diagnosis of CVD and the risk of a subsequent hip fracture [7]. Moreover, male survivors of myocardial infarction have been reported to have low BMD [8]. In addition, significant correlations have been found between osteoporosis and hypertension [14-16], atherosclerosis [17], vascular calcification [18], and congestive heart failure (CHF) [19]. Several CV risk factors, such as physical inactivity, smoking, dyslipidemia, diabetes mellitus, hypertension, oxidative stress, and inflammation have also been associated with a higher incidence of low BMD.

Based on this data, this article is focused on reviewing what is known regarding the relationship and interaction between CVD and osteoporosis including pathophysiological mechanisms, epidemiological aspects, and common risk factors.

2. The Common Risk Factors for Cardiovascular Disease and Osteoporosis

2.1. Hypertension

Hypertension is defined as a condition in which the values of systolic and diastolic blood pressure are higher than 140 mm Hg and 90 mm Hg, respectively [20]. This condition remains the leading cause of death worldwide and is therefore the world's greatest public health problem [21]. Epidemiological studies suggest that elevated blood pressure is an independent predictor of CVD [22]. Both hypertension and osteoporosis are multi-factorial disorders in which genetic and lifestyle factors contribute to pathogenesis [23, 24]. Factors associated with an increase in blood pressure include age, physical inactivity, excessive alcohol use, and excessive salt intake. These same factors also contribute to the risk of developing osteoporosis. [16]

Hypertension itself may be a risk factor for osteoporosis. However, existing evidence regarding the association between high blood pressure and bone loss is inconclusive. In a large cohort of British women, Cappuccio et al. found that femoral neck BMD detected by the dual-energy X-ray absorptiometric (DEXA) method was inversely related to the highest tertile of systolic and diastolic blood pressure values [25]. In contrast, Mussolino et al. reported that there were no significant associations between BMD and hypertension in men or women of African American or white ethnicity using data from the National Health and Nutrition Examination Survey (NHANES) [26]. These conflicting results in previously reported studies may be explained by different patient populations, diagnostic methods, or diagnostic criteria.

Evidence from several animal and clinical studies suggests that high blood pressure is associated with bone metabolism. Specifically, the calcium loss related to high blood pressure may be due to a defect in the ability of the kidney to process calcium which in turn may lead to increased movement of calcium from bone, thereby increasing the risk for osteoporosis. Several studies have consistently reported that a sustained increase in urinary calcium excretion as a result of high blood pressure may be the underlying mechanism [16, 27]. Calcium metabolism has been investigated in patients with essential hypertension and normal renal function to evaluate renal calcium processing and the reported increase in renal calcium loss [27]. These results support the hypothesis of primary renal calcium leak in essential hypertension. Furthermore, hypertension is presumed to be associated with abnormal calcium metabolism leading to increased calcium loss, compensatory activation of the parathyroid gland, and increased movement of calcium from bone [25, 28]. Such long-lasting disturbances in calcium metabolism may constitute one of the mechanisms that contribute to the pathophysiology of hypertensive bone loss.

The renin-angiotensin system (RAS) is an important component of blood pressure regulation. Several epidemiological studies have reported benefits of angiotensin-converting enzyme (ACE) inhibitors (ACEIs) and angiotensin receptor blockers (ARBs) in increasing bone mass and decreasing the risk of bone fractures [29-33]. The main physiological function of both ACEIs and ARBs is blocking the function of angiotensin II. The RAS, from which angiotensin II is synthesized, might be involved in bone metabolism [29, 30]. Animal studies have implicated angiotensin II in the occurrence of osteoporosis [32] and human studies have suggested that increased angiotensin II levels in hypertensive patients have a harmful effect by increasing bone resorption and inhibiting mineralization [34-36]. It has been postulated that angiotensin II plays an important role in hypertension-related osteoporosis, as angiotensin II receptors are expressed in both osteoblasts and osteoclasts [31, 32, 37]. The differentiation of osteoclasts is primarily controlled by the actions of osteoprotegerin (OPG) and the RANKL (receptor activator of nuclear factor κB ligand) system [38-40]. Cbfa1 and RANKL, important factors for maintaining bone homeostasis and key mediators in controlling osteoblast and osteoclast differentiation, are both regulated by cAMP-dependent signaling. Angiotensin II down-regulates the expression of Cbfa1 but up-regulates RANKL expression. By altering the ratio of Cbfa1/RANKL expression via the cAMP-dependent pathway, angiotensin II differently regulates osteoblast and osteoclast differentiation and can lead to enhanced bone resorption and reduced bone formation [41].

2.2. Lipid Metabolism and Osteoporosis

A strong causal relationship between dyslipidemia and CVD has been established based on evidence from animal studies, laboratory investigations, epidemiological studies, and controlled clinical trials [42]. Regarding the close association between osteoporosis and CVD, common mechanisms have been considered as part of a possible relationship between bone loss and lipid disorders. The data concerning relationships between lipid levels and BMD has been inconsistent. Data from several epidemiological and experimental studies suggest that dyslipidemia may play a significant pathogenic role in age-related osteoporosis. The decrease in BMD associated with osteoporosis has been closely related to high lipid levels [43-47]. For example, the levels of serum total cholesterol (TC) and low-density lipoprotein cholesterol (LDL-C) were inversely associated with BMD. Adami et al. also found that total body and hip BMD were positively related to serum triglycerides in women [44]. In contrast, a large population-based observational study from the NHAEMS III survey [48], and a longitudinal analysis from the Framingham study cohort

[49] indicated insignificant direct influences of serum lipids on changes in BMD.

Based on experimental observations, it has been proposed that LDL-C and HDL-C may act on osteoblasts, osteoclasts, and vascular smooth muscle cells [50-53]. Oxidized lipids have been shown to inhibit osteoblastic differentiation in both in vitro [54], and in vivo studies [55]. Because immature osteoblasts are located immediately adjacent to the subendothelial matrix of bone vessels, lipid accumulation in the subendothelial matrix would be expected to inhibit differentiation of these bone-forming cells. In addition, oxidized lipids would be expected to promote bone resorption by recruitment and differentiation of osteoclast precursor cells as oxidized lipids induce endothelial expression of monocyte chemotactic factors and M-CSF, a potent inducer of osteoclastic differentiation.

Moreover, it has been established that the rate of demineralization at the hip is significantly associated with the rate of atherogenesis [56]. The contribution of atherosclerosis is also supported by the observation that arterial disease of the lower limbs may lead to bone mineral loss [57]. Collectively, these observations suggest an indirect role for lipids as linking factors between CVD and osteoporosis via promotion of atherogenesis and arterial stenosis, which in turn may contribute to bone loss, especially at skeletal sites with end-arterial blood supplies.

2.3. Osteoporosis and Vascular Calcification

The association between CVD and vascular calcification was first described in the 19th century [58]. Vascular calcification that can lead to devastating organ dysfunction is commonly seen with aging, end-stage renal disease, diabetes, and atherosclerosis. Calcification of CV structures is associated with arterial stiffness, hypertension, myocardial ischemia, disorders of cardiac valves and CHF. In coronary arteries, calcification is positively correlated with atherosclerotic plaque burden [59, 60], increased risk of myocardial infarction [61], and plaque instability [62]. Vascular calcification has been found to coexist with bone loss in numerous epidemiological studies, suggesting a relationship between both disorders [63-65]. Low BMD is a risk factor for increased mortality later in life, especially from CVD [63]. Results from the population-based Framingham Heart Study cohort indicated that women with the greatest magnitude of bone loss had the most severe progression of abdominal aortic calcification [64]. Aortic calcification is a strong predictor for low BMD and fragility fractures [65].

In the past, vascular calcification was considered a degenerative consequence of aging. It is now understood that calcium deposition in the vasculature is an active and regulated process related to bone formation [66, 67]. However, whether the association between osteoporosis and vascular calcification is causal has not been demonstrated definitively. Bone and vascular tissue share several features at the molecular and cellular levels. OPG, a secreted protein that inhibits osteoclast formation, has been considered a possible link between bone and vascular disease [68]. A subpopulation of artery wall cells in atherosclerotic arteries has the ability to undergo osteoblastic differentiation and may express various bone matrix proteins, including osteopontin [69], osteocalcin [70], matrix vesicles [71], and bone morphogenetic proteins (BMPs) [72]. It has been postulated by Price et al. that bone turnover leading to release of circulating nucleational complexes may explain the link between vascular calcification and osteoporosis in postmenopausal women [73, 74]. In addition, alterations in calcium and phosphorus balance promote bone loss and vascular calcification via multiple mechanisms [75] with calciotropic hormones such as parathyroid hormone and vitamin D playing pivotal roles. Finally, vascular calcification or atherosclerotic disease could decrease peripheral blood supply resulting in bone loss by affecting bone metabolism, suppressing bone cell function, or limiting physical activity.

2.4. Immunological and Inflammatory Factors

A relationship between atherosclerosis markers and bone disease has also been postulated. The association of bone loss with CVD has stimulated a search for common mediators linking the skeletal and vascular systems. Atherosclerotic calcification is a regulated process with many cellular mechanisms similar to bone formation and resorption. Data from epidemiological and clinical studies suggest that atherosclerosis is essentially an inflammatory response to a variety of risk factors and that the consequences of this response may lead to future CV events. Inflammatory cytokines, including interleukin-1, interleukin-6, tumor necrosis factor (TNF), and C-reactive protein (CRP) have been implicated in atherogenesis [76-79]. New insights into the process of bone turnover suggest that inflammation also exerts significant influences on bone physiology and remodeling which can induce osteoporosis [80, 81]. Inflammatory markers associated with atherosclerosis, which also play a role in vascular calcification, have also been shown to predict changes in BMD [82]. The presence of osteoblastic cells in the vascular wall has also been detected [83]. Regulatory proteins produced by bone cells, including osteocalcin, osteopontin, OPG, RANKL, and BMPs are found in atherosclerotic lesions [84], suggesting a regulatory role for these proteins not only in osteoclastogenesis but also in atherosclerotic calcification.

Since its initial discovery as a key regulator in bone metabolism, OPG has become the subject of intense interest for its role in vascular atherosclerosis and calcification. OPG is a protein from the TNF receptor family that regulates the osteoclastogenesis process through inhibition of RANKL, which is a key factor in bone remodeling [85]. It prevents RANKL from binding to its receptor on osteoclasts, thereby inhibiting osteoclastogenesis. It has been reported that OPG is highly expressed in the bones, heart, and major arteries [86]. OPG has been shown not only to be an inhibitor of osteoclastogenesis, but also to be an inflammatory cytokine implicated in arterial calcification, atherosclerosis and CVD [87]. For instance, OPG is up-regulated in calcified coronary plaques and is associated with coronary angiographic disease severity and CV events independent of conventional risk factors [88, 89]. These findings suggest that increased OPG may be a compensatory response to accentuated bone loss and enhanced vascular calcification and that OPG may serve as a marker for both osteoporosis and CVD.

2.5. CHF and Osteoporosis

CHF and osteoporosis are two common chronic conditions in the elderly and both are disabling conditions that adversely affect quality of life due to the associated morbidity and mortality. Many patients with end-stage CVD have risk factors for osteoporosis such as older age and physical inactivity.

In CHF patients, a significant association was found between ejection fraction or CHF severity, as expressed by New York Heart Association (NYHA) function class severity, and frailty score [19]. The reduced BMD in CHF patients may be due to multiple factors. Physical activity is an important determinant of bone health. CHF patients, particularly those who had greater comorbid illness, displayed reduced physical performance, higher disability and higher frailty scores as compared to non-CHF elderly individuals [19]. Physical performance and frailty were associated with lower BMD measurements and vitamin D levels and with higher levels of proinflammatory cytokines [90]. The levels of the inflammatory cytokines, TNF, CRP and IL-6, were significantly increased in CHF patients and were found to be higher in those CHF patients with higher frailty scores [90-93]. In CHF patients, low vitamin D levels may have been attributable to lack of sunlight exposure from immobility, reduced hepatic synthesis of vitamin D, changes in kidney function or impaired intestinal absorption of vitamin D [19]. Vitamin D insufficiency usually results in increased parathyroid hormone (PTH) secretion in order to maintain calcium homeostasis. Interestingly, a relationship between the deteriorating NYHA functional classes in CHF patients with hyperparathyroidism has been reported [94, 95].

3. CV Medicines that Affect Bone

There have been important developments in our understanding of the mechanisms underlying the development of CVD, and several of these mechanisms also underlie osteoporosis. Drugs given to treat CVD may impact bone health in either a beneficial or a harmful way.

3.1. ACEIs/ARBs

The RAS governs body fluid and electrolyte balance and blood pressure [96]. Renin produced by the juxtaglomerular apparatus of the kidney and secreted into the circulation cleaves angiotensinogen to angiotensin I, which is cleaved by ACE to generate angiotensin II. ACEIs act on the crucial enzyme that generates angiotensin II, whereas ARBs act directly on the angiotensin II receptor that responds to angiotensin II stimulation. Blockade of the RAS has been shown to be beneficial in patients with atherosclerosis, hypertension, acute myocardial infarction, chronic systolic heart failure, stroke and diabetic renal disease [97-103].

As discussed previously, the RAS plays an important role in bone metabolism and hypertension-related osteoporosis. It is therefore reasonable to hypothesize that blockade of the RAS may ameliorate osteoporosis and hypertension. Previous animal and epidemiological research reports have described the benefits of ACEIs including increasing bone mass and decreasing the risk for bone fractures [29, 30, 32, 33]. In a cross-sectional study of 3887 elderly Chinese patients, use of ACEIs was associated with higher BMD after adjusting for age, weight, height, thiazide, β-blocker, calcium channel blocker, statin, corticosteroid, and calcium supplement use, history of diabetes, heart disease, peripheral vascular disease, cigarette smoking, alcohol intake, and physical activity level [29]. However, findings regarding the effects of treatment with ARBs on bone mass from animal studies have been inconsistent [31, 32] and the ability of ARBs to modulate bone cell function and reduce fracture incidence in humans has not yet been established. Currently, no clinical trials regarding the effects of ACEIs or ARBs in osteoporosis treatment have been conducted and therefore, there is insufficient evidence to consider blockade of the RAS as a treatment for osteoporosis.

3.2. β-blockers

Experimental evidence suggests that bone remodelling may be partly under the control of the sympathetic nervous system [104-106]. Sympathetic nerve fibers have been discovered in bone and adrenergic receptors in osteoblasts and osteoclasts have been described [105]. One animal study demonstrated leptin-dependent neuronal regulation of bone formation through sympathetic activation with potential therapeutic implications for osteoporosis [106]. The sympathetic nervous system, activated by leptin, can modulate bone resorption through β-adrenergic receptors located in osteoblasts, thus increasing RANKL secretion and resulting in the promotion of osteoclast differentiation [107, 108]. Despite what is known regarding the role of the sympathetic nervous system in regulating bone mass, the ability of β-blockers to modulate bone cell function and reduce fracture incidence in humans has not yet been established.

Not all studies have found a significant association between β-blocker use and fracture. Several observational database and case–control human studies have identified a decreased fracture risk in β-blocker users [33, 109-112]. Other observational studies [113-115] have not found a significant association. The data obtained from the Australian Dubbo Osteoporosis Epidemiology Study (N=3488) demonstrated a significantly lower risk of fractures associated with β-blocker use independent of body mass index (BMI), BMD, age, and other covariates [110]. A large case-control analysis (N=30,601) found that β-blocker use was associated with a significantly lower risk of fractures after adjustment for BMI, smoking status, and the use of other classes of antihypertensives [112]. Results of a meta-analysis of such observational studies, comprising 7 studies of β-blockers, concluded that β-blocker use was associated with a significant decrease in fracture risk. [116]. However, another meta-analysis of fracture incidence in clinical trials of β-blockers for heart failure cast doubt on this finding [117]. Therefore, there is not an adequate evidence base to support using β-blockers as a treatment for osteoporosis, nor can they be regarded as a discriminating risk factor for fracture assessment. It remains unlikely that the current confusing situation will be resolved without definitive, randomized, controlled trials of β-blockers that include fracture as an endpoint.

3.3. Statins

Statins are widely used for the treatment of hypercholesterolemia. They inhibit 3-hydroxy-3-methylglutarylcoenzyme A reductase competitively and reduce hepatic cholesterol synthesis [118]. Statins have both antiatherosclerotic effects and beneficial pleiotropic effects. Consequently, statins reduce the incidence of CVD significantly [119]. In addition, statins may have effects on bone metabolism. A role for statins in bone metabolism was first proposed in 1999, when increased cancellous bone volume was observed in rats treated orally with statins [120]. It has been well established that cholesterol synthesis and osteoclast activation both involve the same biochemical cascade [120-123]. Statins are effective at preventing osteoclast activation by preventing mevalonate production [120]. In turn, bone remodeling is reduced, bone resorption decreases, and the balance of bone resorption and formation is restored. One animal study demonstrated that statins could increase bone formation [22]. Thus, subjects with risk for osteoporosis may benefit from statin therapy.

Several observational population and case–control studies have demonstrated that statin administration was associated with a decreased risk of bone fracture [124-126]. Chan et al. found that statins seemed to be protective against non-pathological fracture among older women [124]. Meier et al. suggested that current exposure to statins was associated with a decreased risk of bone fractures in individuals age 50 years and older [125]. Similarly, an association between statin use by elderly patients and a reduced risk of hip fracture was also reported [126]. However, not all studies demonstrated this association [127-129]. In the United Kingdom, a large case-control analysis (N=163,760) found that use of statins at dosages prescribed in clinical practice was not associated with a reduced risk of fracture [127]. A study of subjects with ischemic heart disease randomly assigned pravastatin or placebo offered no support for the hypothesis that statins had a significant effect on fracture risk [128]. It should be noted, however, that this study did not involve an osteoporotic population.

In summary, a biologically plausible mechanism for statins to affect bone has been asserted and in vitro studies have demonstrated an increase in osteoblast differentiation and bone formation. Prospective randomized controlled trials are needed to better delineate the role of statins in osteoporosis.

3.4. Thiazide Diuretics

Thiazide diuretics remain the most widely used first-line therapy for hypertension [20]. These agents act to inhibit the reabsorption of sodium and chloride and promote calcium reabsorption, resulting in a positive calcium balance which might be expected to have positive effects on BMD.

Not all observational studies have found a significant association between use of thiazide diuretics and fracture [130, 131]. The inconsistent findings could reflect that the protective effect may only manifest after prolonged use and does not persist after cessation of treatment with thiazide diuretics [114, 132-135]. A prospective study in older men and women suggested that the use of thiazide diuretic agents was associated with a reduction of approximately one third in the risk of hip fracture [134]. Schoof et al. suggested that thiazide diuretics protected against hip fracture, but this protective effect disappeared within 4 months after use was discontinued [135]. There have been two prospective randomized trials of thiazide diuretics and BMD. Bolland et al. demonstrated that hydrochlorothiazide treatment in healthy postmenopausal women produced benefits on BMD [136]. LaCroix et al. also found low-dose hydrochlorothiazide preserved BMD in healthy older adults [137].

3.5. Loop Diuretics

Loop diuretics are used mainly in the treatment of fluid overload in CHF. Loop diuretics act to inhibit chloride and sodium reabsorption in the ascending limb of the loop of Henle and also inhibit reabsorption of magnesium and calcium. Reduced renal reabsorption of calcium may be compensated for by increased PTH driving increased synthesis of 1,25-dihdroxyvitamin D and gastrointestinal calcium absorption. This cascade most likely results in a negative effect on bone health [138].

Use of loop diuretics has been identified as a risk factor for low BMD in elderly women [139] and prospective studies have demonstrated increased bone loss at the hip in older men and women [138, 140]. Observational studies have described an association between use of loop diuretics and increased fracture [131, 141]. These results suggest that the potential for bone loss should be considered when loop diuretics are prescribed to older patients in clinical practice.

CONCLUSION

In summary, osteoporosis is associated with hypertension, dyslipidemia, and increased CVD risk, a phenomenon that may be driven by inflammation, atherosclerosis, vascular calcification, and the resulting increase in arterial stiffness. Significant advances have been made in recent years in elucidating the pathophysiological relationship and common risk factors between osteoporosis, fractures, and CVD. Different studies have shown the effect of drugs widely used for CVD, such as statins, and antihypertensives, including ACEIs/ARBs, β-blockers, and thiazide diuretics on bone metabolism. An improved understanding of the pathophysiological mechanisms common to these conditions may contribute to future development of therapies that can act on both bone metabolism and CVD.

REFERENCES

[1] Seeman E, Delmas PD. Bone quality--the material and structural basis of bone strength and fragility. *N Engl J Med.* 2006 May 25;354(21):2250-61.

[2] Warburton DE, Nicol CW, Bredin SS. Health benefits of physical activity: the evidence. *CMAJ.* 2006 Mar 14;174(6):801-9.

[3] Farhat GN, Newman AB, Sutton-Tyrrell K, Matthews KA, Boudreau R, Schwartz AV, Harris T, Tylavsky F, Visser M, Cauley JA; Health ABC Study. The association of bone mineral density measures with incident cardiovascular disease in older adults. *Osteoporos Int.* 2007 Jul;18(7):999-1008.

[4] Kado DM, Browner WS, Blackwell T, Gore R, Cummings SR. Rate of bone loss is associated with mortality in older women: a prospective study. *J Bone Miner Res.* 2000 Oct;15(10):1974-80.

[5] Gupta G, Aronow WS. Atherosclerotic vascular disease may be associated with osteoporosis or osteopenia in postmenopausal women: a preliminary study. *Arch Gerontol Geriatr.* 2006 Sep-Oct;43(2):285-8.

[6] Ness J, Aronow WS. Comparison of prevalence of atherosclerotic vascular disease in postmenopausal women with osteoporosis or osteopenia versus without osteoporosis or osteopenia. *Am J Cardiol.* 2006 May 15;97(10):1427-8.

[7] Sennerby U, Melhus H, Gedeborg R, Byberg L, Garmo H, Ahlbom A, Pedersen NL, Michaëlsson K. Cardiovascular diseases and risk of hip fracture. *JAMA.* 2009 Oct 21;302(15):1666-73.

[8] Magnus JH, Broussard DL. Relationship between bone mineral density and myocardial infarction in US adults. *Osteoporos Int.* 2005 Dec;16(12):2053-62.

[9] Barengolts EI, Berman M, Kukreja SC, Kouznetsova T, Lin C, Chomka EV. Osteoporosis and coronary atherosclerosis in asymptomatic postmenopausal women. *Calcif Tissue Int.* 1998 Mar;62(3):209-13.

[10] Broussard DL, Magnus JH. Coronary heart disease risk and bone mineral density among U.S. women and men. *J Womens Health* (Larchmt). 2008 Apr;17(3):479-90.

[11] Varma R, Aronow WS, Basis Y, Singh T, Kalapatapu K, Weiss MB, Pucillo AL, Monsen CE. Relation of bone mineral density to frequency of coronary heart disease. *Am J Cardiol.* 2008 Apr 15;101(8):1103-4.

[12] Marcovitz PA, Tran HH, Franklin BA, O'Neill WW, Yerkey M, Boura J, Kleerekoper M, Dickinson CZ. Usefulness of bone mineral density to predict significant coronary artery disease. *Am J Cardiol.* 2005 Oct 15;96(8):1059-63.

[13] Erbilen E, Yazici S, Ozhan H, Bulur S, Ordu S, Yazici M. Relationship between angiographically documented coronary artery disease and low bone mass in men. *Circ J.* 2007 Jul;71(7):1095-8.

[14] Woo J, Kwok T, Leung J, Tang N. Dietary intake, blood pressure and osteoporosis. *J Hum Hypertens.* 2009 Jul;23(7):451-5.

[15] Resnick LM, Laragh JH, Sealey JE, Alderman MH. Divalent cations in essential hypertension. Relations between serum ionized calcium, magnesium, and plasma renin activity. *N Engl J Med.* 1983 Oct 13;309(15):888-91.

[16] Cappuccio FP, Kalaitzidis R, Duneclift S, Eastwood JB. Unravelling the links between calcium excretion, salt intake, hypertension, kidney stones and bone metabolism. *J Nephrol.* 2000 May-Jun;13(3):169-77.

[17] Tankò LB, Bagger YZ, Christiansen C. Low bone mineral density in the hip as a marker of advanced atherosclerosis in elderly women. *Calcif Tissue Int.* 2003 Jul;73(1):15-20.

[18] Choi SH, An JH, Lim S, Koo BK, Park SE, Chang HJ, Choi SI, Park YJ, Park KS, Jang HC, Shin CS. Lower bone mineral density is associated with higher coronary calcification and coronary plaque burdens by multidetector row coronary computed tomography in pre- and postmenopausal women. *Clin Endocrinol (Oxf).* 2009 Nov;71(5):644-51.

[19] Abou-Raya S, Abou-Raya A. Osteoporosis and congestive heart failure (CHF) in the elderly patient: double disease burden. *Arch Gerontol Geriatr.* 2009 Sep-Oct;49(2):250-4.

[20] Chobanian AV, Bakris GL, Black HR, Cushman WC, Green LA, Izzo JL Jr, Jones DW, Materson BJ, Oparil S, Wright JT Jr, Roccella EJ; National Heart, Lung, and Blood Institute Joint National Committee on Prevention, Detection, Evaluation, and Treatment of High Blood Pressure; National High Blood Pressure Education Program Coordinating Committee. The Seventh Report of the Joint National Committee on Prevention, Detection, Evaluation, and Treatment of High Blood Pressure: the JNC 7 report. *JAMA.* 2003 May 21;289(19):2560-72.

[21] Murray CJ, Lopez AD. Mortality by cause for eight regions of the world: Global Burden of Disease Study. *Lancet.* 1997 May 3;349(9061):1269-76.

[22] Collins R, Peto R, MacMahon S, Hebert P, Fiebach NH, Eberlein KA, Godwin J, Qizilbash N, Taylor JO, Hennekens CH. Blood pressure, stroke, and coronary heart disease. Part 2, Short-term reductions in blood pressure: overview of randomised drug trials in their epidemiological context. *Lancet.* 1990 Apr 7;335(8693):827-38.

[23] Lifton RP. Molecular genetics of human blood pressure variation. *Science.* 1996 May 3;272(5262):676-80.

[24] Ralston SH, de Crombrugghe B. Genetic regulation of bone mass and susceptibility to osteoporosis. *Genes Dev.* 2006 Sep 15;20(18):2492-506.

[25] Cappuccio FP, Meilahn E, Zmuda JM, Cauley JA. High blood pressure and bone-mineral loss in elderly white women: a prospective study.

Study of Osteoporotic Fractures Research Group. *Lancet.* 1999 Sep 18;354(9183):971-5.

[26] Mussolino ME, Gillum RF. Bone mineral density and hypertension prevalence in postmenopausal women: results from the Third National Health and Nutrition Examination Survey. *Ann Epidemiol.* 2006 May;16(5):395-9.

[27] Strazzullo P, Nunziata V, Cirillo M, Giannattasio R, Ferrara LA, Mattioli PL, Mancini M. Abnormalities of calcium metabolism in essential hypertension. *Clin Sci (Lond).* 1983 Aug;65(2):137-41.

[28] McCarron DA, Pingree PA, Rubin RJ, Gaucher SM, Molitch M, Krutzik S. Enhanced parathyroid function in essential hypertension: a homeostatic response to a urinary calcium leak. *Hypertension.* 1980 Mar-Apr;2(2):162-8.

[29] Lynn H, Kwok T, Wong SY, Woo J, Leung PC. Angiotensin converting enzyme inhibitor use is associated with higher bone mineral density in elderly Chinese. *Bone.* 2006 Apr;38(4):584-8.

[30] Shimizu H, Nakagami H, Osako MK, Nakagami F, Kunugiza Y, Tomita T, Yoshikawa H, Rakugi H, Ogihara T, Morishita R. Prevention of osteoporosis by angiotensin-converting enzyme inhibitor in spontaneous hypertensive rats. *Hypertens Res.* 2009 Sep;32(9):786-90.

[31] Izu Y, Mizoguchi F, Kawamata A, Hayata T, Nakamoto T, Nakashima K, Inagami T, Ezura Y, Noda M. Angiotensin II type 2 receptor blockade increases bone mass. *J Biol Chem.* 2009 Feb 20;284(8):4857-64.

[32] Asaba Y, Ito M, Fumoto T, Watanabe K, Fukuhara R, Takeshita S, Nimura Y, Ishida J, Fukamizu A, Ikeda K. Activation of renin-angiotensin system induces osteoporosis independently of hypertension. *J Bone Miner Res.* 2009 Feb;24(2):241-50.

[33] Rejnmark L, Vestergaard P, Mosekilde L. Treatment with beta-blockers, ACE inhibitors, and calcium-channel blockers is associated with a reduced fracture risk: a nationwide case-control study. *J Hypertens.* 2006 Mar;24(3):581-9.

[34] Pérez-Castrillón JL, Justo I, Silva J, Sanz A, Igea R, Escudero P, Pueyo C, Diaz C, Hernández G, Dueñas A. Bone mass and bone modelling markers in hypertensive postmenopausal women. *J Hum Hypertens.* 2003 Feb;17(2):107-10.

[35] Hatton R, Stimpel M, Chambers TJ. Angiotensin II is generated from angiotensin I by bone cells and stimulates osteoclastic bone resorption in vitro. *J Endocrinol.* 1997 Jan;152(1):5-10.

[36] Hiruma Y, Inoue A, Hirose S, Hagiwara H. Angiotensin II stimulates the proliferation of osteoblast-rich populations of cells from rat calvariae. *Biochem Biophys Res Commun.* 1997 Jan 3;230(1):176-8.

[37] Shimizu H, Nakagami H, Osako MK, Hanayama R, Kunugiza Y, Kizawa T, Tomita T, Yoshikawa H, Ogihara T, Morishita R. Angiotensin II accelerates osteoporosis by activating osteoclasts. *FASEB J.* 2008 Jul;22(7):2465-75.

[38] Teitelbaum SL. Bone resorption by osteoclasts. *Science.* 2000 Sep 1;289(5484):1504-8.

[39] Tintut Y, Parhami F, Tsingotjidou A, Tetradis S, Territo M, Demer LL. 8-Isoprostaglandin E2 enhances receptor-activated NFkappa B ligand (RANKL)-dependent osteoclastic potential of marrow hematopoietic precursors via the cAMP pathway. *J Biol Chem.* 2002 Apr 19;277(16):14221-6.

[40] Tintut Y, Parhami F, Le V, Karsenty G, Demer LL. Inhibition of osteoblast-specific transcription factor Cbfa1 by the cAMP pathway in osteoblastic cells. Ubiquitin/proteasome-dependent regulation. *J Biol Chem.* 1999 Oct 8;274(41):28875-9.

[41] Guan XX, Zhou Y, Li JY. Reciprocal roles of angiotensin II and angiotensin II receptors blockade (ARB) in regulating Cbfa1/RANKL via cAMP signaling pathway: possible mechanism for hypertension-related osteoporosis and antagonistic effect of ARB on hypertension-related osteoporosis. *Int J Mol Sci.* 2011;12(7):4206-13.

[42] Expert Panel on Detection, Evaluation, and Treatment of High Blood Cholesterol in Adults. Executive Summary of The Third Report of The National Cholesterol Education Program (NCEP) Expert Panel on Detection, Evaluation, And Treatment of High Blood Cholesterol In Adults (Adult Treatment Panel III). *JAMA.* 2001 May 16;285(19):2486-97.

[43] Broulik PD, Kapitola J. Interrelations between body weight, cigarette smoking and spine mineral density in osteoporotic Czech women. *Endocr Regul.* 1993 Jun;27(2):57-60.

[44] Adami S, Braga V, Zamboni M, Gatti D, Rossini M, Bakri J, Battaglia E. Relationship between lipids and bone mass in 2 cohorts of healthy women and men. *Calcif Tissue Int.* 2004 Feb;74(2):136-42.

[45] Brownbill RA, Ilich JZ. Lipid profile and bone paradox: higher serum lipids are associated with higher bone mineral density in postmenopausal women. *J Womens Health (Larchmt).* 2006 Apr;15(3):261-70.

[46] Pinals RS, Jabbs JM. Type-IV hyperlipoproteinaemia and transient osteoporosis. *Lancet.* 1972 Oct 28;2(7783):929.

[47] Cui LH, Shin MH, Chung EK, Lee YH, Kweon SS, Park KS, Choi JS. Association between bone mineral densities and serum lipid profiles of pre- and post-menopausal rural women in South Korea. *Osteoporos Int.* 2005 Dec;16(12):1975-81.

[48] Solomon DH, Avorn J, Canning CF, Wang PS. Lipid levels and bone mineral density. *Am J Med.* 2005 Dec;118(12):1414.

[49] Samelson EJ, Cupples LA, Hannan MT, Wilson PW, Williams SA, Vaccarino V, Zhang Y, Kiel DP. Long-term effects of serum cholesterol on bone mineral density in women and men: the Framingham Osteoporosis Study. *Bone.* 2004 Mar;34(3):557-61.

[50] Parhami F, Basseri B, Hwang J, Tintut Y, Demer LL. High-density lipoprotein regulates calcification of vascular cells. *Circ Res.* 2002 Oct 4;91(7):570-6.

[51] Parhami F, Garfinkel A, Demer LL. Role of lipids in osteoporosis. *Arterioscler Thromb Vasc Biol.* 2000 Nov;20(11):2346-8.

[52] Parhami F, Morrow AD, Balucan J, Leitinger N, Watson AD, Tintut Y, Berliner JA, Demer LL. Lipid oxidation products have opposite effects on calcifying vascular cell and bone cell differentiation. A possible explanation for the paradox of arterial calcification in osteoporotic patients. *Arterioscler Thromb Vasc Biol.* 1997 Apr;17(4):680-7.

[53] Tintut Y, Morony S, Demer LL. Hyperlipidemia promotes osteoclastic potential of bone marrow cells ex vivo. *Arterioscler Thromb Vasc Biol.* 2004 Feb;24(2):e6-10.

[54] Parhami F, Jackson SM, Tintut Y, Le V, Balucan JP, Territo M, Demer LL. Atherogenic diet and minimally oxidized low density lipoprotein inhibit osteogenic and promote adipogenic differentiation of marrow stromal cells. *J Bone Miner Res.* 1999 Dec;14(12):2067-78.

[55] Parhami F, Tintut Y, Beamer WG, Gharavi N, Goodman W, Demer LL. Atherogenic high-fat diet reduces bone mineralization in mice. *J Bone Miner Res.* 2001 Jan;16(1):182-8.

[56] Bagger YZ, Tankó LB, Alexandersen P, Qin G, Christiansen C; Prospective Epidemiological Risk Factors Study Group. Radiographic measure of aorta calcification is a site-specific predictor of bone loss and fracture risk at the hip. *J Intern Med.* 2006 Jun;259(6):598-605.

[57] Laroche M, Pouilles JM, Ribot C, Bendayan P, Bernard J, Boccalon H, Mazieres B. Comparison of the bone mineral content of the lower limbs

in men with ischaemic atherosclerotic disease. *Clin Rheumatol.* 1994 Dec;13(4):611-4.

[58] Virchow R. Cellular pathology. As based upon physiological and pathological histology. Lecture XVI--Atheromatous affection of arteries. 1858. *Nutr Rev.* 1989 Jan;47(1):23-5.

[59] Rumberger JA, Simons DB, Fitzpatrick LA, Sheedy PF, Schwartz RS. Coronary artery calcium area by electron-beam computed tomography and coronary atherosclerotic plaque area. A histopathologic correlative study. *Circulation.* 1995 Oct 15;92(8):2157-62.

[60] Sangiorgi G, Rumberger JA, Severson A, Edwards WD, Gregoire J, Fitzpatrick LA, Schwartz RS. Arterial calcification and not lumen stenosis is highly correlated with atherosclerotic plaque burden in humans: a histologic study of 723 coronary artery segments using nondecalcifying methodology. *J Am Coll Cardiol.* 1998 Jan;31(1):126-33.

[61] Loecker TH, Schwartz RS, Cotta CW, Hickman JR Jr. Fluoroscopic coronary artery calcification and associated coronary disease in asymptomatic young men. *J Am Coll Cardiol.* 1992 May;19(6):1167-72.

[62] Fitzgerald PJ, Ports TA, Yock PG. Contribution of localized calcium deposits to dissection after angioplasty. An observational study using intravascular ultrasound. *Circulation.* 1992 Jul;86(1):64-70.

[63] von der Recke P, Hansen MA, Hassager C. The association between low bone mass at the menopause and cardiovascular mortality. *Am J Med.* 1999 Mar;106(3):273-8.

[64] Kiel DP, Kauppila LI, Cupples LA, Hannan MT, O'Donnell CJ, Wilson PW. Bone loss and the progression of abdominal aortic calcification over a 25 year period: the Framingham Heart Study. *Calcif Tissue Int.* 2001 May;68(5):271-6.

[65] Schulz E, Arfai K, Liu X, Sayre J, Gilsanz V. Aortic calcification and the risk of osteoporosis and fractures. *J Clin Endocrinol Metab.* 2004 Sep;89(9):4246-53.

[66] Doherty TM, Asotra K, Fitzpatrick LA, Qiao JH, Wilkin DJ, Detrano RC, Dunstan CR, Shah PK, Rajavashisth TB. Calcification in atherosclerosis: bone biology and chronic inflammation at the arterial crossroads. *Proc Natl Acad Sci U S A.* 2003 Sep 30;100(20):11201-6.

[67] Abedin M, Tintut Y, Demer LL. Vascular calcification: mechanisms and clinical ramifications. *Arterioscler Thromb Vasc Biol.* 2004 Jul;24(7):1161-70.

[68] Bucay N, Sarosi I, Dunstan CR, Morony S, Tarpley J, Capparelli C, Scully S, Tan HL, Xu W, Lacey DL, Boyle WJ, Simonet WS. osteoprotegerin-deficient mice develop early onset osteoporosis and arterial calcification. *Genes Dev.* 1998 May 1;12(9):1260-8.
[69] Giachelli CM, Bae N, Almeida M, Denhardt DT, Alpers CE, Schwartz SM. Osteopontin is elevated during neointima formation in rat arteries and is a novel component of human atherosclerotic plaques. *J Clin Invest.* 1993 Oct;92(4):1686-96.
[70] Levy RJ, Schoen FJ, Levy JT, Nelson AC, Howard SL, Oshry LJ. Biologic determinants of dystrophic calcification and osteocalcin deposition in glutaraldehyde-preserved porcine aortic valve leaflets implanted subcutaneously in rats. *Am J Pathol.* 1983 Nov;113(2):143-55.
[71] Tanimura A, McGregor DH, Anderson HC. Matrix vesicles in atherosclerotic calcification. *Proc Soc Exp Biol Med.* 1983 Feb;172(2):173-7.
[72] Boström K, Watson KE, Horn S, Wortham C, Herman IM, Demer LL. Bone morphogenetic protein expression in human atherosclerotic lesions. *J Clin Invest.* 1993 Apr;91(4):1800-9.
[73] Price PA, Caputo JM, Williamson MK. Bone origin of the serum complex of calcium, phosphate, fetuin, and matrix Gla protein: biochemical evidence for the cancellous bone-remodeling compartment. *J Bone Miner Res.* 2002 Jul;17(7):1171-9.
[74] Price PA, Faus SA, Williamson MK. Bisphosphonates alendronate and ibandronate inhibit artery calcification at doses comparable to those that inhibit bone resorption. *Arterioscler Thromb Vasc Biol.* 2001 May;21(5):817-24.
[75] Giachelli CM. Vascular calcification mechanisms. *J Am Soc Nephrol.* 2004 Dec;15(12):2959-64.
[76] Libby P, Simon DI. Inflammation and thrombosis: the clot thickens. *Circulation.* 2001 Apr 3;103(13):1718-20.
[77] Libby P, Ridker PM. Novel inflammatory markers of coronary risk: theory versus practice. *Circulation.* 1999 Sep 14;100(11):1148-50.
[78] Devaraj S, Xu DY, Jialal I. C-reactive protein increases plasminogen activator inhibitor-1 expression and activity in human aortic endothelial cells: implications for the metabolic syndrome and atherothrombosis. *Circulation.* 2003 Jan 28;107(3):398-404.

[79] Pasceri V, Willerson JT, Yeh ET. Direct proinflammatory effect of C-reactive protein on human endothelial cells. *Circulation.* 2000 Oct 31;102(18):2165-8.

[80] Arron JR, Choi Y. Bone versus immune system. *Nature.* 2000 Nov 30;408(6812):535-6.

[81] Lorenzo J. Interactions between immune and bone cells: new insights with many remaining questions. *J Clin Invest.* 2000 Sep;106(6):749-52.

[82] Ding C, Parameswaran V, Udayan R, Burgess J, Jones G. Circulating levels of inflammatory markers predict change in bone mineral density and resorption in older adults: a longitudinal study. *J Clin Endocrinol Metab.* 2008 May;93(5):1952-8.

[83] Watson KE, Boström K, Ravindranath R, Lam T, Norton B, Demer LL. TGF-beta 1 and 25-hydroxycholesterol stimulate osteoblast-like vascular cells to calcify. *J Clin Invest.* 1994 May;93(5):2106-13.

[84] Dhore CR, Cleutjens JP, Lutgens E, Cleutjens KB, Geusens PP, Kitslaar PJ, Tordoir JH, Spronk HM, Vermeer C, Daemen MJ. Differential expression of bone matrix regulatory proteins in human atherosclerotic plaques. A*rterioscler Thromb Vasc Biol.* 2001 Dec;21(12):1998-2003.

[85] Schoppet M, Preissner KT, Hofbauer LC. RANK ligand and osteoprotegerin: paracrine regulators of bone metabolism and vascular function. *Arterioscler Thromb Vasc Biol.* 2002 Apr 1;22(4):549-53.

[86] Simonet WS, Lacey DL, Dunstan CR, Kelley M, Chang MS, Lüthy R, Nguyen HQ, Wooden S, Bennett L, Boone T, Shimamoto G, DeRose M, Elliott R, Colombero A, Tan HL, Trail G, Sullivan J, Davy E, Bucay N, Renshaw-Gegg L, Hughes TM, Hill D, Pattison W, Campbell P, Sander S, Van G, Tarpley J, Derby P, Lee R, Boyle WJ. Osteoprotegerin: a novel secreted protein involved in the regulation of bone density. *Cell.* 1997 Apr 18;89(2):309-19.

[87] McFarlane SI, Muniyappa R, Shin JJ, Bahtiyar G, Sowers JR. Osteoporosis and cardiovascular disease: brittle bones and boned arteries, is there a link? *Endocrine.* 2004 Feb;23(1):1-10.

[88] Kiechl S, Schett G, Wenning G, Redlich K, Oberhollenzer M, Mayr A, Santer P, Smolen J, Poewe W, Willeit J. Osteoprotegerin is a risk factor for progressive atherosclerosis and cardiovascular disease. *Circulation.* 2004 May 11;109(18):2175-80.

[89] Jono S, Ikari Y, Shioi A, Mori K, Miki T, Hara K, Nishizawa Y. Serum osteoprotegerin levels are associated with the presence and severity of coronary artery disease. *Circulation.* 2002 Sep 3;106(10):1192-4.

[90] Walston J, McBurnie MA, Newman A, Tracy RP, Kop WJ, Hirsch CH, Gottdiener J, Fried LP; Cardiovascular Health Study. Frailty and activation of the inflammation and coagulation systems with and without clinical comorbidities: results from the Cardiovascular Health Study. *Arch Intern Med.* 2002 Nov 11;162(20):2333-41.

[91] Cesari M, Penninx BW, Newman AB, Kritchevsky SB, Nicklas BJ, Sutton-Tyrrell K, Tracy RP, Rubin SM, Harris TB, Pahor M. Inflammatory markers and cardiovascular disease (The Health, Aging and Body Composition [Health ABC] Study). *Am J Cardiol.* 2003 Sep 1;92(5):522-8.

[92] Wei J, Xu H, Davies JL, Hemmings GP. Increase of plasma IL-6 concentration with age in healthy subjects. *Life Sci.* 1992;51(25):1953-6.

[93] Reuben DB, Cheh AI, Harris TB, Ferrucci L, Rowe JW, Tracy RP, Seeman TE. Peripheral blood markers of inflammation predict mortality and functional decline in high-functioning community-dwelling older persons. *J Am Geriatr Soc.* 2002 Apr;50(4):638-44.

[94] Garakyaraghi M, Kerdegari M, Siavash M. Calcium and vitamin D status in heart failure patients in Isfahan, Iran. *Biol Trace Elem Res.* 2010 Jun;135(1-3):67-73.

[95] Bozic B, Loncar G, Prodanovic N, Lepic T, Radojicic Z, Cvorovic V, Dimkovic S, Popovic V. Parathyroid hormone response to vitamin D insufficiency in elderly males with chronic heart failure. *Physiol Res.* 2011;60 Suppl 1:S155-63.

[96] Peach MJ. Renin-angiotensin system: biochemistry and mechanisms of action. *Physiol Rev.* 1977 Apr;57(2):313-70.

[97] Julius S, Kjeldsen SE, Weber M, Brunner HR, Ekman S, Hansson L, Hua T, Laragh J, McInnes GT, Mitchell L, Plat F, Schork A, Smith B, Zanchetti A; VALUE trial group. Outcomes in hypertensive patients at high cardiovascular risk treated with regimens based on valsartan or amlodipine: the VALUE randomised trial. *Lancet.* 2004 Jun 19;363(9426):2022-31.

[98] Dahlöf B, Devereux RB, Kjeldsen SE, Julius S, Beevers G, de Faire U, Fyhrquist F, Ibsen H, Kristiansson K, Lederballe-Pedersen O, Lindholm LH, Nieminen MS, Omvik P, Oparil S, Wedel H; LIFE Study Group. Cardiovascular morbidity and mortality in the Losartan Intervention For Endpoint reduction in hypertension study (LIFE): a randomised trial against atenolol. *Lancet.* 2002 Mar 23;359(9311):995-1003.

[99] Hansson L, Lindholm LH, Ekbom T, Dahlöf B, Lanke J, Scherstén B, Wester PO, Hedner T, de Faire U. Randomised trial of old and new antihypertensive drugs in elderly patients: cardiovascular mortality and morbidity the Swedish Trial in Old Patients with Hypertension-2 study. *Lancet.* 1999 Nov 20;354(9192):1751-6.
[100] Hansson L, Lindholm LH, Niskanen L, Lanke J, Hedner T, Niklason A, Luomanmäki K, Dahlöf B, de Faire U, Mörlin C, Karlberg BE, Wester PO, Björck JE. Effect of angiotensin-converting-enzyme inhibition compared with conventional therapy on cardiovascular morbidity and mortality in hypertension: the Captopril Prevention Project (CAPPP) randomised trial. *Lancet.* 1999 Feb 20;353(9153):611-6.
[101] Yusuf S, Sleight P, Pogue J, Bosch J, Davies R, Dagenais G. Effects of an angiotensin-converting-enzyme inhibitor, ramipril, on cardiovascular events in high-risk patients. The Heart Outcomes Prevention Evaluation Study Investigators. *N Engl J Med.* 2000 Jan 20;342(3):145-53.
[102] Jamerson K, Weber MA, Bakris GL, Dahlöf B, Pitt B, Shi V, Hester A, Gupte J, Gatlin M, Velazquez EJ; ACCOMPLISH Trial Investigators. Benazepril plus amlodipine or hydrochlorothiazide for hypertension in high-risk patients. *N Engl J Med.* 2008 Dec 4;359(23):2417-28.
[103] Bulpitt CJ, Beckett NS, Cooke J, Dumitrascu DL, Gil-Extremera B, Nachev C, Nunes M, Peters R, Staessen JA, Thijs L; Hypertension in the Very Elderly Trial Working Group. Results of the pilot study for the Hypertension in the Very Elderly Trial. *J Hypertens.* 2003 Dec;21(12):2409-17.
[104] Yadav VK, Oury F, Suda N, Liu ZW, Gao XB, Confavreux C, Klemenhagen KC, Tanaka KF, Gingrich JA, Guo XE, Tecott LH, Mann JJ, Hen R, Horvath TL, Karsenty G. A serotonin-dependent mechanism explains the leptin regulation of bone mass, appetite, and energy expenditure. *Cell.* 2009 Sep 4;138(5):976-89.
[105] Togari A. Adrenergic regulation of bone metabolism: possible involvement of sympathetic innervation of osteoblastic and osteoclastic cells. *Microsc Res Tech.* 2002 Jul 15;58(2):77-84.
[106] Takeda S, Elefteriou F, Levasseur R, Liu X, Zhao L, Parker KL, Armstrong D, Ducy P, Karsenty G. Leptin regulates bone formation via the sympathetic nervous system. *Cell.* 2002 Nov 1;111(3):305-17.
[107] Moore RE, Smith CK 2nd, Bailey CS, Voelkel EF, Tashjian AH Jr. Characterization of beta-adrenergic receptors on rat and human osteoblast-like cells and demonstration that beta-receptor agonists can

stimulate bone resorption in organ culture. *Bone Miner.* 1993 Dec;23(3):301-15.

[108] Elefteriou F, Ahn JD, Takeda S, Starbuck M, Yang X, Liu X, Kondo H, Richards WG, Bannon TW, Noda M, Clement K, Vaisse C, Karsenty G. Leptin regulation of bone resorption by the sympathetic nervous system and CART. *Nature.* 2005 Mar 24;434(7032):514-20.

[109] Pasco JA, Henry MJ, Sanders KM, Kotowicz MA, Seeman E, Nicholson GC; Geelong Osteoporosis Study. Beta-adrenergic blockers reduce the risk of fracture partly by increasing bone mineral density: Geelong Osteoporosis Study. *J Bone Miner Res.* 2004 Jan;19(1):19-24.

[110] Yang S, Nguyen ND, Center JR, Eisman JA, Nguyen TV. Association between beta-blocker use and fracture risk: the Dubbo Osteoporosis Epidemiology Study. *Bone.* 2011 Mar 1;48(3):451-5.

[111] de Vries F, Souverein PC, Cooper C, Leufkens HG, van Staa TP. Use of beta-blockers and the risk of hip/femur fracture in the United Kingdom and The Netherlands. *Calcif Tissue Int.* 2007 Feb;80(2):69-75.

[112] Schlienger RG, Kraenzlin ME, Jick SS, Meier CR. Use of beta-blockers and risk of fractures. *JAMA.* 2004 Sep 15;292(11):1326-32.

[113] Levasseur R, Dargent-Molina P, Sabatier JP, Marcelli C, Bréart G. Beta-blocker use, bone mineral density, and fracture risk in older women: results from the Epidemiologie de l'Osteoporose prospective study. *J Am Geriatr Soc.* 2005 Mar;53(3):550-2.

[114] Solomon DH, Mogun H, Garneau K, Fischer MA. Risk of fractures in older adults using antihypertensive medications. *J Bone Miner Res.* 2011 Jul;26(7):1561-7.

[115] Reid IR, Gamble GD, Grey AB, Black DM, Ensrud KE, Browner WS, Bauer DC. beta-Blocker use, BMD, and fractures in the study of osteoporotic fractures. *J Bone Miner Res.* 2005 Apr;20(4):613-8.

[116] Wiens M, Etminan M, Gill SS, Takkouche B. Effects of antihypertensive drug treatments on fracture outcomes: a meta-analysis of observational studies. *J Intern Med.* 2006 Oct;260(4):350-62.

[117] Reid IR. Effects of beta-blockers on fracture risk. *J Musculoskelet Neuronal Interact.* 2008 Apr-Jun;8(2):105-10.

[118] Endo A. The discovery and development of HMG-CoA reductase inhibitors. *J Lipid Res.* 1992 Nov;33(11):1569-82.

[119] Vaughan CJ, Gotto AM Jr, Basson CT. The evolving role of statins in the management of atherosclerosis. *J Am Coll Cardiol.* 2000 Jan;35(1):1-10.

[120] Mundy G, Garrett R, Harris S, Chan J, Chen D, Rossini G, Boyce B, Zhao M, Gutierrez G. Stimulation of bone formation in vitro and in rodents by statins. *Science.* 1999 Dec 3;286(5446):1946-9.

[121] Fisher JE, Rogers MJ, Halasy JM, Luckman SP, Hughes DE, Masarachia PJ, Wesolowski G, Russell RG, Rodan GA, Reszka AA. Alendronate mechanism of action: geranylgeraniol, an intermediate in the mevalonate pathway, prevents inhibition of osteoclast formation, bone resorption, and kinase activation in vitro. *Proc Natl Acad Sci U S A.* 1999 Jan 5;96(1):133-8.

[122] 122. Luckman SP, Hughes DE, Coxon FP, Graham R, Russell G, Rogers MJ. Nitrogen-containing bisphosphonates inhibit the mevalonate pathway and prevent post-translational prenylation of GTP-binding proteins, including Ras. *J Bone Miner Res.* 1998 Apr;13(4):581-9.

[123] Russell RG, Rogers MJ, Frith JC, Luckman SP, Coxon FP, Benford HL, Croucher PI, Shipman C, Fleisch HA. The pharmacology of bisphosphonates and new insights into their mechanisms of action. *J Bone Miner Res.* 1999 Oct;14 Suppl 2:53-65.

[124] Chan KA, Andrade SE, Boles M, Buist DS, Chase GA, Donahue JG, Goodman MJ, Gurwitz JH, LaCroix AZ, Platt R. Inhibitors of hydroxymethylglutaryl-coenzyme A reductase and risk of fracture among older women. *Lancet.* 2000 Jun 24;355(9222):2185-8.

[125] Meier CR, Schlienger RG, Kraenzlin ME, Schlegel B, Jick H. HMG-CoA reductase inhibitors and the risk of fractures. *JAMA.* 2000 Jun 28;283(24):3205-10.

[126] Wang PS, Solomon DH, Mogun H, Avorn J. HMG-CoA reductase inhibitors and the risk of hip fractures in elderly patients. *JAMA.* 2000 Jun 28;283(24):3211-6.

[127] van Staa TP, Wegman S, de Vries F, Leufkens B, Cooper C. Use of statins and risk of fractures. *JAMA.* 2001 Apr 11;285(14):1850-5.

[128] Reid IR, Hague W, Emberson J, Baker J, Tonkin A, Hunt D, MacMahon S, Sharpe N. Effect of pravastatin on frequency of fracture in the LIPID study: secondary analysis of a randomised controlled trial. Long-term Intervention with Pravastatin in Ischaemic Disease. *Lancet.* 2001 Feb 17;357(9255):509-12.

[129] Pedersen TR, Kjekshus J. Statin drugs and the risk of fracture. 4S Study Group. *JAMA.* 2000 Oct 18;284(15):1921-2.

[130] Cauley JA, Cummings SR, Seeley DG, Black D, Browner W, Kuller LH, Nevitt MC. Effects of thiazide diuretic therapy on bone mass,

fractures, and falls. The Study of Osteoporotic Fractures Research Group. *Ann Intern Med.* 1993 May 1;118(9):666-73.
[131] Heidrich FE, Stergachis A, Gross KM. Diuretic drug use and the risk for hip fracture. *Ann Intern Med.* 1991 Jul 1;115(1):1-6.
[132] Ray WA, Griffin MR, Downey W, Melton LJ 3rd. Long-term use of thiazide diuretics and risk of hip fracture. *Lancet.* 1989 Apr 1;1(8640):687-90.
[133] Felson DT, Sloutskis D, Anderson JJ, Anthony JM, Kiel DP. Thiazide diuretics and the risk of hip fracture. Results from the Framingham Study. *JAMA.* 1991 Jan 16;265(3):370-3.
[134] LaCroix AZ, Wienpahl J, White LR, Wallace RB, Scherr PA, George LK, Cornoni-Huntley J, Ostfeld AM. Thiazide diuretic agents and the incidence of hip fracture. *N Engl J Med.* 1990 Feb 1;322(5):286-90.
[135] Schoofs MW, van der Klift M, Hofman A, de Laet CE, Herings RM, Stijnen T, Pols HA, Stricker BH. Thiazide diuretics and the risk for hip fracture. *Ann Intern Med.* 2003 Sep 16;139(6):476-82.
[136] Bolland MJ, Ames RW, Horne AM, Orr-Walker BJ, Gamble GD, Reid IR. The effect of treatment with a thiazide diuretic for 4 years on bone density in normal postmenopausal women. *Osteoporos Int.* 2007 Apr;18(4):479-86.
[137] LaCroix AZ, Ott SM, Ichikawa L, Scholes D, Barlow WE. Low-dose hydrochlorothiazide and preservation of bone mineral density in older adults. A randomized, double-blind, placebo-controlled trial. *Ann Intern Med.* 2000 Oct 3;133(7):516-26.
[138] Rejnmark L, Vestergaard P, Heickendorff L, Andreasen F, Mosekilde L. Effects of long-term treatment with loop diuretics on bone mineral density, calcitropic hormones and bone turnover. *J Intern Med.* 2005 Feb;257(2):176-84.
[139] Ooms ME, Lips P, Van Lingen A, Valkenburg HA. Determinants of bone mineral density and risk factors for osteoporosis in healthy elderly women. *J Bone Miner Res.* 1993 Jun;8(6):669-75.
[140] Lim LS, Fink HA, Kuskowski MA, Taylor BC, Schousboe JT, Ensrud KE; Osteoporotic Fractures in Men (MrOS) Study Group. Loop diuretic use and increased rates of hip bone loss in older men: the Osteoporotic Fractures in Men Study. *Arch Intern Med.* 2008 Apr 14;168(7):735-40.
[141] Tromp AM, Ooms ME, Popp-Snijders C, Roos JC, Lips P. Predictors of fractures in elderly women. *Osteoporos Int.* 2000;11(2):134-40.

In: Bone Loss
Editor: Kuo-Cheng Lu
ISBN: 978-1-62417-169-7

Chapter 4

BONE LOSS IN MEN WITH PROSTATE CANCER: RISK FACTORS, DETECTION, AND PREVENTION

***Fred Saad*[1], *Karim Fizazi*[2] *and Carsten Goessl*[3]**
[1]University of Montreal Hospital Center, Montreal, QC, Canada,
[2]Institut Gustave Roussy, University of Paris Sud, Villejuif, France,
[3]Amgen Inc., Thousand Oaks, CA, US

ABSTRACT

Prostate cancer is one of the most common cancer types in men in Western countries. In 2008 it was estimated that nearly 900,000 men were diagnosed with prostate cancer worldwide. Prostate cancer typically starts as a localized disease, progressing to nearby tissues (eg, seminal vesicles), before metastasizing to distant sites such as the skeleton. Growth of prostate cancer is fueled by testosterone. Androgen-deprivation therapy (ADT) is used to treat men with both locally advanced disease as well as men with metastatic disease. ADT is effective for slowing the growth of prostate cancer, but it can also lead to substantial bone loss with a resulting increase in fracture risk. There are a number of additional risk factors in this patient population that may further contribute to bone loss and fracture risk. These include low weight, smoking, alcohol consumption, and other co-morbid conditions and medications. In general, bone loss and osteoporosis in older men, even those treated with ADT, is underdiagnosed and, thus, undertreated.

Several tools are available for detection of bone loss or assessment of fracture risk. These include dual-energy X-ray absorptiometry (DXA), FRAX®, an online fracture risk assessment tool incorporating clinically determined risk factors that can be used in combination with DXA results, and measurement of biochemical markers of bone turnover. While multiple options are available for treating bone loss, only denosumab (Prolia®; 60 mg every 6 months SC) is approved to increase bone mass and reduce the risk of fracture in that population. In this review we will discuss (i) the prostate cancer disease course, (ii) ADT and other risk factors for bone loss in this patient population, (iii) tools available to the clinician for detection of bone loss; and (iv) treatment options for bone loss.

INTRODUCTION

Prostate cancer is the most common cancer in the United States with an annual incidence of new cases slightly exceeding those of breast and lung cancer [1]. In 2012, 241,740 new cases are anticipated in the United States out of 848,170 total new cases of all cancer types in men (28.5% of all cancers in men). Just over 28,000 deaths from prostate cancer are expected in 2012, compared to almost 88,000 for men with lung cancer. These statistics reflect the nature of prostate cancer as a chronic disease and highlight the necessity of adopting strategies to control the burden of disease during a prolonged management course.

In the early, organ-confined stages of prostate cancer, active surveillance is an option [2]. Depending on the stage of the clinically localized cancer and expected survival of the patient, radiation, brachytherapy, or radical prostatectomy, with or without pelvic lymph node dissection, may be recommended. A scheme showing a typical natural history of prostate cancer transitioning through various disease states is shown in Figure 1. As the growth of prostate cancer is stimulated by testosterone, androgen deprivation therapy (ADT) with either gonadotropin-releasing hormone agonists or bilateral orchiectomy is the mainstay of therapy for advanced stages [2]. ADT is also frequently used as adjuvant therapy for those with locally advanced cancer undergoing radiation, or following radical prostatectomy, as well as in those with rising PSA subsequent to a primary treatment [3]. Following initial ADT therapy, prostate cancer usually becomes castration-resistant after a variable time period, and ADT is continued at this stage in accordance with guidelines [2]. Eventually metastasis occurs, predominantly to the skeleton, which may lead to skeletal-related events. The focus of the present review is bone loss related to prostate cancer and ADT; bone metastases constitute a separate condition for which established treatments have been defined to prevent the resulting skeletal complications [76, *might also add Saad et al., JNCI 2002*]..

ADT has been shown to improve survival in defined settings [4, 5]. In approximately half of incident prostate cancer cases, patients are treated with ADT [6] and an estimated 1 million prostate cancer survivors worldwide are chemically or surgically castrated [7]. ADT is associated with a number of side effects, including an increased risk for cardiovascular disease, diabetes, sexual dysfunction, hot flashes, gynecomastia, cognitive dysfunction, body composition changes, and exaggerated bone loss with resulting increased fracture risk [8, 9]. Other side effects from ADT, such as sarcopenia and frailty might also contribute to increased fracture risk [10, 11], but are not the focus of this chapter.

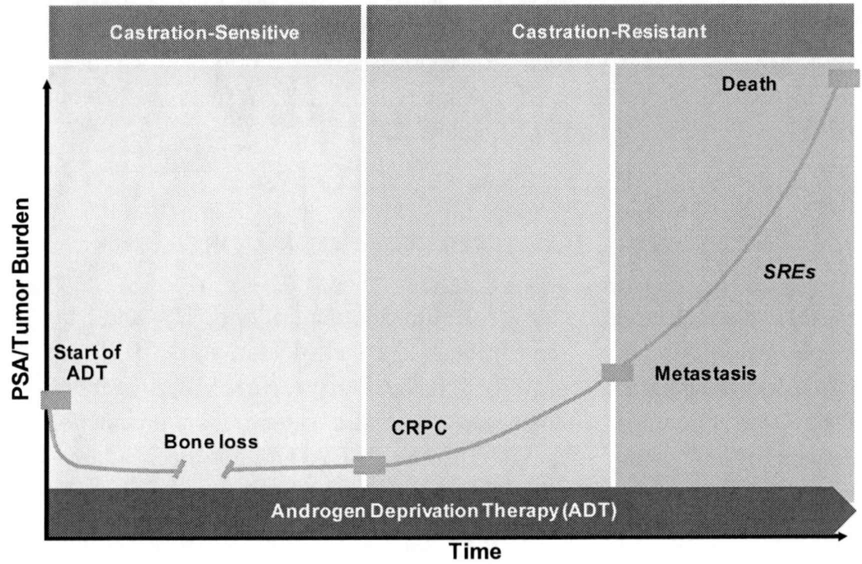

Figure 1. Prostate cancer disease progression and use of androgen-deprivation therapy. PSA, prostate-specific antigen; ADT, androgen deprivation therapy;CRPC, castration-resistant prostate cancer; SREs, skeletal-related events.

Even in the absence of ADT, patients with prostate cancer have a high incidence of osteoporosis, ranging from 33%-63% across several studies [12-15], and exceeding that of age-matched controls (42% in 174 patients vs 27%

in 106 controls, P=0.022) [16]. Additionally, fracture rates in men with prostate cancer not treated with ADT were elevated relative to those expected for the population (15-year cumulative fracture incidence of 44% vs 33% expected, P<0.001)[17]. The etiology of bone loss in non-castrate patients with prostate cancer may be related to the presence of shared risk factors for prostate cancer and osteoporosis, such as vitamin D deficiency or low dietary calcium intake [18].

Though common, bone loss in men is often underdiagnosed and as a result, undertreated. Even in men with prostate cancer, bone mineral density (BMD) testing is rare: a retrospective study in 33,036 men with prostate cancer initiating ADT between 1995 and 2008 in Ontario Canada showed that only 4.8% had a prior BMD test [19]. The rate of BMD testing after initiation of ADT increased substantially over the observation period, but was still under 20 per 100 patient-years in 2008. Further, in a population study including 7339 elderly Caucasian men and 3545 elderly African American men not receiving ADT, <3% and 0% respectively of those with a FRAX® 10-year hip fracture risk of ≥ 3% (National Osteoporosis Foundation recommended intervention threshold [20]) actually received osteoporosis medication [21]. Even in those with hip fractures (n=3347; 96.5% men), only 14.5% received osteoporosis medication within 12 months of fracture [22].

Risk Factors for Bone Loss

ADT is a major risk factor for the development of bone loss and its effects on bone resorption, BMD, and fracture are well-documented. BMD loss has been reported to range from 3-10% in the first year of ADT treatment, thus ADT-related bone loss in men may be more severe than postmenopausal osteoporosis in women [23, 24]. The risks of ADT have been addressed in large systematic reviews including a report in 116,911 patients with prostate cancer showing that patients on ADT had a 30% increased risk of osteoporosis and 17% increased risk of fracture (both P<0.00001) [25]. Similarly, an analysis of the Surveillance Epidemiology and End Results database including 50,613 men with prostate cancer who survived at least 5 years after diagnosis, found a rate of fracture of 19.4% in those receiving ADT versus 12.6% in those who did not (P<0.001) [26]. Other studies have reported that ADT increases fracture risk by 1.7 fold [27].

In addition to ADT, there are a number of other common risk factors for bone loss in men. These include lower weight or weight loss [28, 29], advancing age [29], race (Caucasian) [30, 31], hypogonadism, use of corticosteroids (used in combination with some chemotherapy regimens in prostate cancer and in autoimmune conditions), and use of other immunosuppressive drugs. In particular, bone loss and fractures in patients with rheumatoid arthritis taking glucocorticoids have been well-documented [32, 33]. Modifiable factors such as smoking, excessive alcohol consumption, diet, and low physical activity are other well-known clinical factors associated with bone loss [29, 34-36]. Previous fracture is also an important risk factor for osteoporosis and fracture in both men and women. Poor physical performance has been correlated with low BMD and poor bone microarchitecture [37]. Other co-morbid conditions/medications that could further contribute to bone loss and increase fracture risk include COPD or asthma, gastrointestinal disease, hypercalciuria, hyperthyroidism, hyperparathyroidism, homocystinuria, ankylosing spondylitis, use of anticonvulsant medications, and use of proton pump inhibitors for acid-related gastrointestinal disorders [38, 39]

In an effort to understand the reasons for underdiagnosis of osteoporosis in men, Nelson et al [40] evaluated the risk factors that triggered osteoporosis diagnosis or treatment. The strongest predictors of identification of osteoporosis by primary care physicians were gonadotropin-releasing hormone exposure, rheumatoid arthritis, and fragility fractures, while known clinical factors such as excessive alcohol consumption and smoking were ignored. Thus greater attention to the full spectrum of risk factors could improve the identification and treatment of those at risk for bone loss and fracture.

DETECTION OF BONE LOSS IN MEN

Dual-energy X-ray absorptiometry (DXA) is the most widely used method for the measurement of BMD and is the reference standard for the diagnosis of osteoporosis used by the WHO. Osteoporosis in men is defined by the same WHO criteria as in women: a T-score of $\leq$ -2.5 at the lumbar spine, femoral neck, or total hip. However, it is noteworthy that the relationship between BMD and fracture risk is less well-studied in men than in women. DXA is also an important tool for monitoring the response to osteoporosis treatment. Changes to US Medicare reimbursement in 2007 have resulted in substantial reductions in the use of DXA testing for diagnosis of osteoporosis and for monitoring of treatment [41-43]. Even prior to the reimbursement changes, DXA was underused in men undergoing ADT: in a retrospective study of 184 patients receiving goserelin for at least one year, only 8.7% had received a DXA scan in the past 3 years [44]. In a Canadian study of women with osteoporosis, DXA testing mediated access to treatment, with 34% of those who had undergone DXA testing receiving treatment compared to only 2% in those without DXA testing [45]. Hence the reimbursement-driven reduction in DXA testing is likely to result in increased numbers of patients with osteoporosis failing to receive access to diagnosis and treatment [46].

The FRAX® tool is a World Health Organization (WHO) algorithm designed to predict a patient's 10-year probability of developing a hip fracture or major osteoporotic fracture in patients not previously treated for bone loss [47, 48]. The tool uses the risk factors of age, sex, weight and height, previous fracture, history of hip fracture in a parent, current smoking, glucocorticoid use, rheumatoid arthritis, secondary osteoporosis risk factors (such as hypogonadism, parathyroidism, vitamin D deficiency, etc), and consumption of >3 alcoholic drinks per day. All of these factors are readily obtainable from a patient's medical history. FRAX® does not require BMD, though BMD can be entered if desired. The National Osteoporosis Foundation recommends initiating treatment if the FRAX®-determined 10-year fracture risk is ≥ 3% for hip and ≥ 20% for major osteoporotic fractures [20]. Using the FRAX® tool, over 50% of 363 men with prostate cancer receiving ADT were shown to have a fracture risk sufficient to initiate treatment [49], higher than that predicted by those with a BMD score of -2.5 alone. Older age was highly predictive of fracture risk such that 76.6% of men in their 70s and 98.8% of those over 80 reached the treatment threshold. However the effectiveness of FRAX® in predicting fracture in men with prostate cancer has not been specifically studied in prospective trials. FRAX® may in some cases underestimate the need for treatment: in a recent study in men on ADT for prostate cancer, FRAX® evaluation resulted in underqualification for treatment in patients who were discovered to have spinal fracture on spinal x-rays [50].

In patients with prostate cancer, particularly those receiving ADT, bone loss results in increased serum and urine levels of bone turnover markers, which are degradation products of bone metabolism. Levels of these bone turnover markers can be measured and monitored longitudinally, potentially providing insight into changes in skeletal metabolism [51-53]. Anabolic or bone formation markers include serum osteocalcin, serum procollagen I carboxyterminal propeptide (PICP), serum procollagen type 1 N-terminal propeptide (PINP), bone-specific alkaline phosphatase, and bone sialoprotein. Catabolic or bone resorption markers include serum C-telopeptide [CTX], urinary N-telopeptide [NTX]), serum and urinary hydroxyproline, urinary and urinary-free total pyridinoline (Pyr) and deoxypyridinoline (dPyr), serum carboxyterminal telopeptide of type I collagen (ITCP), and tartrate-resistant acid phosphatase (TRAP or TRACP). In the setting of bone metastatic disease, levels of NTX and CTX have shown associations with both the severity of metastatic disease and the response to treatment [51, 52]. In randomly selected men over age 65, the highest quartile of PINP concentration was associated with a higher rate of bone loss at the total hip, but was not independently associated with hip fracture risk [54]. Such studies have not yet been reported in men with prostate cancer receiving ADT. At the present time, the use of bone turnover markers is largely restricted to clinical trials in which these markers are used to measure the population response to agents for the treatment of bone loss. Information on bone turnover markers can provide a complement to measurement of BMD, particularly since BMD changes occur slowly, whereas in contrast, bone turnover markers may provide a more sensitive means of detecting shorter-term changes in bone metabolism. Use of these markers is currently being validated in clinical trials, and the National Osteoporosis Foundation guidelines state that currently available bone turnover marker tests may not be sufficiently sensitive to measure small responses in individual patients [20].

Currently, DXA BMD measurements provide the most reliable means of both diagnosing bone loss and measuring the response to treatment. However, BMD measurements alone may not be sufficient to adequately predict fracture risk; therefore, use of the FRAX® tool can offer additional guidance. FRAX® offers a useful tool in targeting patients who can most benefit from treatment, but cannot be used to monitor response. Although bone markers are currently considered investigational, they may eventually offer a potentially sensitive and non-invasive means of measuring response, and may offer an additional means of monitoring patients in combination with, or instead of, DXA.

Prevention of Bone Loss

Men with prostate cancer initiating ADT should receive regular BMD evaluations and treatment interventions where warranted: baseline DXA scans should be conducted at ADT initiation with follow-up scans every 1-2 years [55]. Early intervention to prevent bone loss is critical. Based on known risk factors as detailed above, patients should be encouraged to maintain a healthy weight, exercise, take calcium and vitamin D supplementation, and to avoid alcohol consumption and smoking [56-59]. Although some meta-analyses have shown a modest impact of dietary calcium and vitamin D supplementation on reduction of bone loss [60, 61] and fracture risk [62] in elderly non-oncologic populations, these supplements are insufficient to halt bone loss during ADT as observed in the placebo arms of clinical trials in which all patients were to receive calcium and vitamin D supplementation [63-65].

Several therapeutic options are available for the treatment of bone loss and/or for fracture prevention in men with prostate cancer. The National Osteoporosis Foundation and The National Comprehensive Cancer Network (NCCN) guidelines recommend that treatment be considered when the 10-year probability of hip fracture is ≥ 3% or the 10-year probability of major osteoporotic fracture is ≥ 20% [2, 20]. Recommended treatments include denosumab, IV zoledronic acid, and oral alendronate [2]. Denosumab (Prolia®, Amgen; 60 mg every 6 months SC) is the only approved treatment for bone loss in men with nonmetastatic cancer receiving ADT that has been shown to be effective for fracture prevention [65]. Several bisphosphonates including zoledronic acid, risedronate, pamidronate, and alendronate have been shown to increase BMD in this population [64, 66-72] but no trial of bisphosphonates has been adequately powered to demonstrate fracture reduction in this population prospectively. Raloxifene and toremifene, selective estrogen receptor modulators, have been shown to increase BMD in men with prostate cancer on ADT, and toremifene also reduced fracture risk in a phase 3 trial [73]. The future of toremifene for this indication is currently unclear due a Complete Response for Non-Approval letter from the FDA [74].

Denosumab is a subcutaneously administered fully human monoclonal antibody against RANK Ligand (RANKL), the key mediator of osteoclast formation, survival, and function [75]. In the double-blind, placebo-controlled hormone-ablation bone loss trial (HALT), denosumab was evaluated in 1468 men with prostate cancer receiving ADT who were deemed to be at high risk of fracture based on previous osteoporotic fracture, low BMD, and/or age ≥ 70 years [65]. After 24 months of treatment, relative to placebo, denosumab increased BMD by 6.7% at the lumbar spine (primary endpoint), 4.8% at the total hip, 3.9% at the femoral neck, and 5.5% at the distal radius (all $P<0.001$). Significant differences between the treatment groups were observed as early as one month and increased continually over 3 years showing the rapid and sustained action of denosumab. At 36 months, denosumab reduced the risk of vertebral fracture by 62% (1.5% vs 3.9%; relative risk = 0.38, 95% confidence interval, 0.19 – 0.78; $P<0.006$) [65]. This agent is the only one for which prospectively evaluated fracture data are available for men on ADT. The incidence of adverse events was similar between the groups. A higher incidence of cataracts was reported for the denosumab-treated patients in this trial. However, in subsequent trials, including those with over 12-fold the dose intensity used in this trial, no difference in the rate of cataracts has been reported between denosumab-treated patients and the control-group patients [76, 77]. Denosumab is approved in the United States and Europe as a treatment to improve bone mass in men at high risk for fracture receiving ADT.

Bisphosphonates are antiresorptive agents available in both oral and intravenous forms that inhibit osteoclast activity through a distinct mechanism distinct from that of denosumab. While zoledronic acid is approved for male osteoporosis, there are currently no data available from randomized controlled trials to support the effectiveness of bisphosphonates in fracture prevention in men with prostate cancer receiving ADT. A recent meta-analysis including 2634 patients from 15 randomized controlled trials evaluated the effects of bisphosphonates relative to placebo including zoledronic acid (1056 patients from 8 studies), pamidronate (208 patients in 3 studies), clodronate, (275 patients from 2 studies), alendronate (81 patients from 2 studies), and neridronate (15 patients in 1 study) [78]. In this analysis, bisphosphonates were associated with reduced risk for fracture (risk ratio, 0.80; P=0.005) and osteoporosis (RR, 0.39; P<0.00001), and increased BMD relative to placebo by 5.2% at the lumbar spine and 2.4% at the femoral neck. Of note, however, this meta-analysis was dominated by patients with bone metastases and results should be interpreted with caution. In the setting of bone metastases, denosumab 120 mg every 4 weeks SC has been proven superior to IV zoledronic acid 4 mg every 4 weeks in preventing skeletal-related events [76].

CONCLUSION

Although ADT is central to treating high risk and advanced prostate cancers and has resulted in significantly improved outcomes, it is important to recognize that bone health may be compromised in a significant proportion of patients on long-term continuous ADT. In patients with non-metastatic prostate cancer, there are relatively simple tools to help identify those at higher risk of fractures. Effective therapies are now available that may significantly reduce the risk of bone loss and fractures. Screening for bone loss and metastases and early intervention in those at high risk may significantly reduce the risk of complications and maintain quality of life. In the presence of bone metastases and extremely rapid bone turnover, dosing and scheduling of bone targeted therapy increases for maximum efficacy, but the goal essentially remains the same: maintaining bone health and reducing the risk of serious complications.

Acknowledgments

Wanda J.Krall, PhD, a consultant supported by Amgen and Amy K. Foreman-Wykert, PhD (Amgen Inc.) provided writing assistance.

References

[1] Siegel R, Naishadham D, Jemal A. Cancer statistics, 2012. *CA Cancer J Clin.* 2012 Jan-Feb;62(1):10-29.

[2] http://www.nccn.org/professionals/physician_gls/pdf/prostate.pdf. *National Compre-hensive Cancer Center Clinical Practice Guidelines TM Prostate Cancer. Version* 12012. accessed 21 Feb 2012.

[3] Sharifi N, Gulley JL, Dahut WL. Androgen deprivation therapy for prostate cancer. *JAMA.* 2005 Jul 13;294(2):238-44.

[4] Bolla M, Collette L, Blank L, Warde P, Dubois JB, Mirimanoff RO, et al. Long-term results with immediate androgen suppression and external irradiation in patients with locally advanced prostate cancer (an EORTC study): a phase III randomised trial. *Lancet.* 2002 Jul 13;360(9327):103-6.

[5] Messing EM, Manola J, Sarosdy M, Wilding G, Crawford ED, Trump D. Immediate hormonal therapy compared with observation after radical prostatectomy and pelvic lymphadenectomy in men with node-positive prostate cancer. *N Engl J Med.* 1999 Dec 9;341(24):1781-8.

[6] Gilbert SM, Kuo YF, Shahinian VB. Prevalent and incident use of androgen deprivation therapy among men with prostate cancer in the United States. *Urol Oncol.* 2011 Nov;29(6):647-53.

[7] Langley R, Price P, Pollock P, Abel PD. Osteoporosis in patients with prostate cancer on long-term androgen deprivation therapy: an increasing but under-recognised problem. *BJU Int.* 2010 Sep;106(5):726-7; author reply 7.

[8] Smith MR. Androgen deprivation therapy for prostate cancer: new concepts and concerns. *Curr Opin Endocrinol Diabetes Obes.* 2007 Jun;14(3):247-54.

[9] Freedland SJ, Eastham J, Shore N. Androgen deprivation therapy and estrogen deficiency induced adverse effects in the treatment of prostate cancer. *Prostate Cancer Prostatic Dis.* 2009;12(4):333-8.

[10] Bylow K, Mohile SG, Stadler WM, Dale W. Does androgen-deprivation therapy accelerate the development of frailty in older men with prostate cancer?: a conceptual review. *Cancer.* 2007 Dec 15;110(12):2604-13.

[11] Isbarn H, Boccon-Gibod L, Carroll PR, Montorsi F, Schulman C, Smith MR, et al. Androgen deprivation therapy for the treatment of prostate cancer: consider both benefits and risks. *Eur Urol.* 2009 Jan;55(1):62-75.

[12] Agarwal MM, Mandal AK, Khandelwal N, Singh SK. Need for measurement of bone mineral density in patients of prostate cancer before and after orchidectomy: role of quantitative computer tomography. *J Assoc Physicians India.* 2007 Jul;55:486-90.

[13] Morote J, Morin JP, Orsola A, Abascal JM, Salvador C, Trilla E, et al. Prevalence of osteoporosis during long-term androgen deprivation therapy in patients with prostate cancer. *Urology.* 2007 Mar;69(3):500-4.

[14] Wadhwa VK, Weston R, Mistry R, Parr NJ. Long-term changes in bone mineral density and predicted fracture risk in patients receiving androgen-deprivation therapy for prostate cancer, with stratification of treatment based on presenting values. *BJU Int.* 2009 Sep;104(6):800-5.

[15] Smith MR, McGovern FJ, Fallon MA, Schoenfeld D, Kantoff PW, Finkelstein JS. Low bone mineral density in hormone-naive men with prostate carcinoma. *Cancer.* 2001 Jun 15;91(12):2238-45.

[16] Hussain SA, Weston R, Stephenson RN, George E, Parr NJ. Immediate dual energy X-ray absorptiometry reveals a high incidence of osteoporosis in patients with advanced prostate cancer before hormonal manipulation. *BJU Int.* 2003 Nov;92(7):690-4.

[17] Melton LJ, 3rd, Lieber MM, Atkinson EJ, Achenbach SJ, Zincke H, Therneau TM, et al. Fracture risk in men with prostate cancer: a population-based study. *J Bone Miner Res.* 2011 Aug;26(8):1808-15.

[18] Saad F. Bone loss in prostate cancer: evaluation, treatment and prevention. *Can J Urol.* 2005 Feb;12 Suppl 1:71-6; discussion 99-100.

[19] Alibhai SM, Yun L, Cheung AM, Paszat L. Screening for osteoporosis in men receiving androgen deprivation therapy. *JAMA.* 2012 Jan 18;307(3):255-6.

[20] http://www.nof.org/professionals/clinical-guidelines. *National Osteoporosis Foundation Clinical Guidelines.* Accessed 05 March 2012.

[21] Curtis JR, McClure LA, Delzell E, Howard VJ, Orwoll E, Saag KG, et al. Population-based fracture risk assessment and osteoporosis treatment disparities by race and gender. *J Gen Intern Med.* 2009 Aug;24(8):956-62.

[22] Shibli-Rahhal A, Vaughan-Sarrazin MS, Richardson K, Cram P. Testing and treatment for osteoporosis following hip fracture in an integrated U.S. healthcare delivery system. *Osteoporos Int.* 2011 Dec;22(12):2973-80.

[23] Oefelein MG, Resnick MI. The impact of osteoporosis in men treated for prostate cancer. *Urol Clin North Am.* 2004 May;31(2):313-9.

[24] Smith MR. Osteoporosis during androgen deprivation therapy for prostate cancer. *Urology.* 2002 Sep;60(3 Suppl 1):79-85; discussion 6.

[25] Serpa Neto A, Tobias-Machado M, Esteves MA, Senra MD, Wroclawski ML, Fonseca FL, et al. A systematic review and meta-analysis of bone metabolism in prostate adenocarcinoma. *BMC Urol.* 2010;10:9.

[26] Shahinian VB, Kuo YF, Freeman JL, Goodwin JS. Risk of fracture after androgen deprivation for prostate cancer. *N Engl J Med.* 2005 Jan 13;352(2):154-64.

[27] Lau YK, Lee E, Prior HJ, Lix LM, Metge CJ, Leslie WD. Fracture risk in androgen deprivation therapy: a Canadian population based analysis. *Can J Urol.* 2009 Dec;16(6):4908-14.

[28] Thomas-John M, Codd MB, Manne S, Watts NB, Mongey AB. Risk factors for the development of osteoporosis and osteoporotic fractures among older men. *J Rheumatol.* 2009 Sep;36(9):1947-52.

[29] Papaioannou A, Kennedy CC, Cranney A, Hawker G, Brown JP, Kaiser SM, et al. Risk factors for low BMD in healthy men age 50 years or older: a systematic review. *Osteoporos Int.* 2009 Apr;20(4):507-18.

[30] Saylor PJ, Morton RA, Hancock ML, Barnette KG, Steiner MS, Smith MR. Factors associated with vertebral fractures in men treated with androgen deprivation therapy for prostate cancer. *J Urol.* 2011 Aug;186(2):482-6.

[31] Morgans AK, Hancock ML, Barnette KG, Steiner MS, Morton RA, Smith MR. Racial differences in bone mineral density and fractures in men receiving androgen deprivation therapy for prostate cancer. *J Urol.* 2012 Mar;187(3):889-93.

[32] Weinstein RS. Glucocorticoid-induced osteonecrosis. *Endocrine.* 2011 Dec 15.

[33] Baker JF, George M, Baker DG, Toedter G, Von Feldt JM, Leonard MB. Associations between body mass, radiographic joint damage, adipokines and risk factors for bone loss in rheumatoid arthritis. *Rheumatology* (Oxford). 2011 Nov;50(11):2100-7.

[34] Langsetmo L, Hitchcock CL, Kingwell EJ, Davison KS, Berger C, Forsmo S, et al. Physical activity, body mass index and bone mineral density-associations in a prospective population-based cohort of women and men: the Canadian Multicentre Osteoporosis Study (CaMos). *Bone.* 2012 Jan;50(1):401-8.

[35] Yan C, Avadhani NG, Iqbal J. The effects of smoke carcinogens on bone. *Curr Osteoporos Rep.* 2011 Dec;9(4):202-9.

[36] Ronis MJ, Mercer K, Chen JR. Effects of nutrition and alcohol consumption on bone loss. *Curr Osteoporos Rep.* 2011 Jun;9(2):53-9.

[37] Blaizot S, Boutroy S, Vilayphiou N, Boonen S, Chapurlat R, Szulc P. Poor bone microarchitecture in older men with impaired physical performance-the STRAMBO study. *Osteoporos Int.* 2012 Jan 31.

[38] Ngamruengphong S, Leontiadis GI, Radhi S, Dentino A, Nugent K. Proton pump inhibitors and risk of fracture: a systematic review and meta-analysis of observational studies. *Am J Gastroenterol.* 2011 Jul;106(7):1209-18; quiz 19.

[39] http://www.niams.nih.gov/Health_Info/Bone/Osteoporosis/men.asp. *NIH Osteoporsis and Related Bone Diseases National Resource Center.* Accessed 05 March 2012.

[40] Nelson RE, Nebeker JR, Sauer BC, Lafleur J. Factors associated with screening or treatment initiation among male United States veterans at risk for osteoporosis fracture. *Bone.* 2012 Jan 18.

[41] O'Malley CD, Johnston SS, Lenhart G, Cherkowski G, Palmer L, Morgan SL. Trends in dual-energy X-ray absorptiometry in the United States, 2000-2009. *J Clin Densitom.* 2011 Apr-Jun;14(2):100-7.

[42] King AB, Fiorentino DM. Medicare payment cuts for osteoporosis testing reduced use despite tests' benefit in reducing fractures. *Health Aff (Millwood).* 2011 Dec;30(12):2362-70.

[43] Zhang J, Delzell E, Zhao H, Laster AJ, Saag KG, Kilgore ML, et al. Central DXA utilization shifts from office-based to hospital-based settings among medicare beneficiaries in the wake of reimbursement changes. *J Bone Miner Res.* 2011 Dec 20.

[44] Tanvetyanon T. Physician practices of bone density testing and drug prescribing to prevent or treat osteoporosis during androgen deprivation therapy. *Cancer.* 2005 Jan 15;103(2):237-41.

[45] Cadarette SM, Gignac MA, Jaglal SB, Beaton DE, Hawker GA. Access to osteoporosis treatment is critically linked to access to dual-energy x-ray absorptiometry testing. *Med Care.* 2007 Sep;45(9):896-901.

[46] Tanner SB. Dual-energy X-ray absorptiometry in clinical practice: new guidelines and concerns. *Curr Opin Rheumatol.* 2011 Jul;23(4):385-8.

[47] http://www.shef.ac.uk/FRAX. *FRAX WHO Fracture Risk Assessment Tool.* Accessed 05 March 2012.

[48] Kanis JA, Oden A, Johansson H, Borgstrom F, Strom O, McCloskey E. FRAX and its applications to clinical practice. *Bone.* 2009 May;44(5):734-43.

[49] Saylor PJ, Kaufman DS, Michaelson MD, Lee RJ, Smith MR. Application of a fracture risk algorithm to men treated with androgen deprivation therapy for prostate cancer. *J Urol.* 2010 Jun;183(6):2200-5.

[50] Neubecker K, Adams-Huet B, Farukhi IM, Delapena RC, Gruntmanis U. Predictors of fracture risk and bone mineral density in men with prostate cancer on androgen deprivation therapy. *J Osteoporos.* 2011;2011:924595.

[51] Saad F, Eastham JA, Smith MR. Biochemical markers of bone turnover and clinical outcomes in men with prostate cancer. *Urol Oncol.* 2010 Dec 15.

[52] Lipton A, Costa L, Coleman RE. Bone turnover markers: Tools for prognosis and monitoring response to bisphosphonates? *Breast Dis.* 2011 Dec 5.

[53] Garnero P. Markers of bone turnover in prostate cancer. *Cancer Treat Rev.* 2001 Jun;27(3):187-92; discussion 93-6.

[54] Bauer DC, Garnero P, Harrison SL, Cauley JA, Eastell R, Ensrud KE, et al. Biochemical markers of bone turnover, hip bone loss, and fracture in older men: the MrOS study. *J Bone Miner Res.* 2009 Dec;24(12):2032-8.

[55] Saad F, Adachi JD, Brown JP, Canning LA, Gelmon KA, Josse RG, et al. Cancer treatment-induced bone loss in breast and prostate cancer. *J Clin Oncol.* 2008 Nov 20;26(33):5465-76.

[56] Lee CE, Leslie WD, Czaykowski P, Gingerich J, Geirnaert M, Lau YK. A comprehensive bone-health management approach for men with prostate cancer receiving androgen deprivation therapy. *Curr Oncol.* 2011 Aug;18(4):e163-72.

[57] Tipples K, Robinson A. Optimal management of cancer treatment-induced bone loss: considerations for elderly patients. *Drugs Aging.* 2011 Nov 1;28(11):867-83.

[58] Grossmann M, Hamilton EJ, Gilfillan C, Bolton D, Joon DL, Zajac JD. Bone and metabolic health in patients with non-metastatic prostate cancer who are receiving androgen deprivation therapy. *Med J Aust.* 2011 Mar 21;194(6):301-6.

[59] Daniell HW. Osteoporosis due to androgen deprivation therapy in men with prostate cancer. *Urology.* 2001 Aug;58(2 Suppl 1):101-7.

[60] Daly RM, Brown M, Bass S, Kukuljan S, Nowson C. Calcium- and vitamin D3-fortified milk reduces bone loss at clinically relevant skeletal sites in older men: a 2-year randomized controlled trial. *J Bone Miner Res.* 2006 Mar;21(3):397-405.

[61] Dawson-Hughes B, Harris SS, Krall EA, Dallal GE. Effect of calcium and vitamin D supplementation on bone density in men and women 65 years of age or older. *N Engl J Med.* 1997 Sep 4;337(10):670-6.

[62] Tang BM, Eslick GD, Nowson C, Smith C, Bensoussan A. Use of calcium or calcium in combination with vitamin D supplementation to prevent fractures and bone loss in people aged 50 years and older: a meta-analysis. *Lancet.* 2007 Aug 25;370(9588):657-66.

[63] Michaelson MD, Kaufman DS, Lee H, McGovern FJ, Kantoff PW, Fallon MA, et al. Randomized controlled trial of annual zoledronic acid to prevent gonadotropin-releasing hormone agonist-induced bone loss in men with prostate cancer. *J Clin Oncol.* 2007 Mar 20;25(9):1038-42.

[64] Smith MR, Eastham J, Gleason DM, Shasha D, Tchekmedyian S, Zinner N. Randomized controlled trial of zoledronic acid to prevent bone loss in men receiving androgen deprivation therapy for nonmetastatic prostate cancer. *J Urol.* 2003 Jun;169(6):2008-12.

[65] Smith MR, Egerdie B, Hernandez Toriz N, Feldman R, Tammela TL, Saad F, et al. Denosumab in men receiving androgen-deprivation therapy for prostate cancer. *N Engl J Med.* 2009 Aug 20;361(8):745-55.

[66] Taxel P, Dowsett R, Richter L, Fall P, Klepinger A, Albertsen P. Risedronate prevents early bone loss and increased bone turnover in the first 6 months of luteinizing hormone-releasing hormone-agonist therapy for prostate cancer. *BJU Int.* 2010 Nov;106(10):1473-6.

[67] Izumi K, Mizokami A, Sugimoto K, Narimoto K, Kitagawa Y, Koh E, et al. Risedronate prevents persistent bone loss in prostate cancer patients treated with androgen deprivation therapy: results of a 2-year follow-up study. *Prostate Cancer Prostatic Dis.* 2011 Sep;14(3):238-42.

[68] Rodrigues P, Meler A, Hering F. Titration of dosage for the protective effect of zoledronic acid on bone loss in patients submitted to androgen deprivation therapy due to prostate cancer: a prospective open-label study. *Urol Int.* 2010;85(2):180-5.

[69] Ryan CW, Huo D, Demers LM, Beer TM, Lacerna LV. Zoledronic acid initiated during the first year of androgen deprivation therapy increases bone mineral density in patients with prostate cancer. *J Urol.* 2006 Sep;176(3):972-8; discussion 8.

[70] Smith MR, McGovern FJ, Zietman AL, Fallon MA, Hayden DL, Schoenfeld DA, et al. Pamidronate to prevent bone loss during androgen-deprivation therapy for prostate cancer. *N Engl J Med.* 2001 Sep 27;345(13):948-55.

[71] Israeli RS, Rosenberg SJ, Saltzstein DR, Gottesman JE, Goldstein HR, Hull GW, et al. The effect of zoledronic acid on bone mineral density in patients undergoing androgen deprivation therapy. *Clin Genitourin Cancer.* 2007 Mar;5(4):271-7.

[72] Greenspan SL, Nelson JB, Trump DL, Resnick NM. Effect of once-weekly oral alendronate on bone loss in men receiving androgen deprivation therapy for prostate cancer: a randomized trial. *Ann Intern Med.* 2007 Mar 20;146(6):416-24.

[73] Smith MR, Malkowicz SB, Brawer MK, Hancock ML, Morton RA, Steiner MS. Toremifene decreases vertebral fractures in men younger than 80 years receiving androgen deprivation therapy for prostate cancer. *J Urol.* 2011 Dec;186(6):2239-44.

[74] http://www.news-medical.net/news/20091102/FDA-issues-a-Complete-Response-Letter-for-GTx-toremifene-NDA.aspx. *FDA Issues a Complete Response Letter for GTx Toremifene.* Accessed 05 March 2012.

[75] Lacey DL, Timms E, Tan HL, Kelley MJ, Dunstan CR, Burgess T, et al. Osteoprotegerin ligand is a cytokine that regulates osteoclast differentiation and activation. *Cell.* 1998 Apr 17;93(2):165-76.

[76] Fizazi K, Carducci M, Smith M, Damiao R, Brown J, Karsh L, et al. Denosumab versus zoledronic acid for treatment of bone metastases in men with castration-resistant prostate cancer: a randomised, double-blind study. *Lancet.* 2011 Mar 5;377(9768):813-22.

[77] Smith MR, Saad F, Coleman R, Shore N, Fizazi K, Tombal B, et al. Denosumab and bone-metastasis-free survival in men with castration-resistant prostate cancer: results of a phase 3, randomised, placebo-controlled trial. *Lancet.* 2012 Jan 7;379(9810):39-46.

[78] Serpa Neto A, Tobias-Machado M, Esteves MA, Senra MD, Wroclawski ML, Fonseca FL, et al. Bisphosphonate therapy in patients under androgen deprivation therapy for prostate cancer: a systematic review and meta-analysis. *Prostate Cancer Prostatic Dis.* 2012 Mar;15(1):36-44.

In: Bone Loss
Editor: Kuo-Cheng Lu
ISBN: 978-1-62417-169-7

Chapter 5

HYPERPROLACTINEMIA AS A RISK FACTOR FOR BONE LOSS

Erika C. O. Naliato
Serra dos Órgãos University Center, Teresópolis/RJ, Brazil

ABSTRACT

Prolactin (PRL) is a peptide hormone produced mainly by the pituitary gland. Hyperprolactinemia can be physiological, pathological or pharmacological. Patients with hyperprolactinemia are susceptible to developing osteopenia and osteoporosis. The secondary hypogonadism seems to be responsible for bone loss in patients with hyperprolactinemia. The degree of bone loss is proportional to the duration of hyperprolactinemia and its consequent hypogonadism. The hyperprolactinemia-related bone loss can be severe, especially in children and adolescents, since it can restrict peak bone mass acquisition. Although men are generally less prone to developing osteoporosis, those with hyperprolactinemia are as equally affected as women by bone loss. The skeletal site which is the most frequently affected by hyperprolactinemia is the lumbar spine. This site is formed basically by trabecular bone, which is especially affected by hormonal disturbances such as hyperprolactinemia and hypogonadism. Bone loss can be reversed or at least interrupted once adequate levels of gonadal steroids and PRL are established.

Abbreviations

AR: Androgen receptor
BMD: Bone mineral density
CAP: Cyclase activating fraction of parathormone
CIP: Cyclase inhibiting fraction of parathormone
CTx: C-terminal telopeptide of type I collagen
DA-2: Dopamine receptor(s) type 2
DHT: Dihydrotestosterone
ER: Estrogen receptor
GnRH: Gonadotropin-releasing hormone
IGF-1: Insulin-like growth factor
IL-6: Interleukin-6
mRNA: Messenger ribonucleic acid
OPG: Osteoprotegerin
PRL: Prolactin
PTH: Parathormone
PTHrP: Parathormone-related peptide
RANKL: Receptor activator of nuclear factor kB ligand
RUNX2: Runt-related transcription factor 2
SD: Standard-deviation
SHBG: Sex hormones-binding globulin
TGF-beta: Transforming growth factor-beta

Introduction

Prolactin (PRL) is a peptide hormone produced essentially by the pituitary gland [1]. The main physiological role of PRL is the stimulation of the production of milk by the mammary glands [2,3]. Hypothalamic factors are responsible for the regulation of PRL production and release by the anterior pituitary [2,3]. Dopamine is the dominant factor involved in the regulation of PRL secretion, exerting an inhibitory control of its production and release [2,3]. As a consequence, in men and non-pregnant women, PRL secretion is usually maintained and continuously inhibited [2,3].

Hyperprolactinemia consists of a persistent elevation of serum PRL levels and is the most frequent disorder of the hypothalamic-pituitary axis. Increased PRL levels may be physiological (for example, gestation and lactation), pathological or pharmacological. The main pathological cause of hyperprolactinemia is the prolactinoma, a pituitary tumor that produces PRL. In addition, drugs such as antipsychotic agents, selective serotonin reuptake inhibitors, and estrogens can increase PRL secretion by the anterior pituitary and lead to hyperprolactinemia [3]. Clinical manifestations of hyperprolactinemia include galactorrhea, headaches and, when it leads to secondary hypogonadism, which is frequent, it can also incur in menstrual irregularity, loss of libido, and impotence [3,4,5]. Women are significantly more affected by hyperprolactinemia than men [3,4].

Hyperprolactinemia is a very common endocrine disorder and it is estimated that 48% of the individuals affected by hyperprolactinemia develop osteopenia or osteoporosis [6]. In these patients, bone loss indexes may reach 10 to 30% at the lumbar spine [6, 7, 8, 9, 10, 11, 12], 5 to 8% at the radius [7,8], 15% at the femoral neck [11,12,13], and approximately 11% at the trochanter [6].

Two main mechanisms have been suggested to be responsible for hyperprolactinemia-induced bone loss: (1) secondary hypogonadism and (2) a direct effect of PRL on bone. The hyperprolactinemic bone loss is progressive [14,15] but the process may be interrupted by the reversal of the hyperprolactinemic status [7,8,16,17].

This chapter will discuss the importance of hyperprolactinemia as a risk factor for bone loss, the pathophysiology of hyperprolactinemia-induced bone loss, and the influence of the appropriate treatment of hyperprolactinemia and secondary hypogonadism on the reversal of bone loss and stabilization of bone mass.

Pathophysiology of Hyperprolactinemia-Induced Bone Loss

Hypogonadism

Situations characterized by hypogonadism, such as athletes' amenorrhea, anorexia nervosa, hypothalamic amenorrhea, and menopause are frequently associated with increased bone resorption and consequent reduction of bone mineral density (BMD) [18,19,20,21]. Even relatively small deficits of estradiol and testosterone in women with regular menses may compromise BMD [22,23]. Slemenda et al. (1996) studied the consequences of hypogonadism on bone metabolism and concluded that, in premenopausal women, bone loss is particularly associated with low levels of androgens, while during menopause either low levels of androgens or estrogens might induce bone loss [22]. Additional studies developed with postmenopausal women have demonstrated that estrogen replacement therapy is capable of inhibiting bone loss when adequate serum concentrations of sex steroids are achieved [24]. In female athletes, vertebral BMD has been found to be significantly related to menstrual patterns [18].

Hyperprolactinemia can cause hypogonadism through the suppression of the hypothalamic-pituitary-gonadal axis. This process may affect both men and women [25,26,27]. The prevalence of hypogonadism among women and men with hyperprolactinemia is high [5,11,14,28,29,30,31].

Animal models of hyperprolactinemia reinforce the role of hypogonadism on bone loss [32]. Additionally, in women with hyperprolactinemia, secondary hypogonadism seems to be the main responsible for the decrease in bone mass [33,34]. These data were reinforced by studies that demonstrated that women with hyperprolactinemia-induced amenorrhea tend to present osteopenia [10,14,15,31,35,36,37], while hyperprolactinemic women who do not develop amenorrhea are not subjected to BMD reduction[15,33,34,37]. Furthermore, in women with prolactinoma, a direct correlation between the annual frequency of menstrual cycles and BMD has been established [10].

Although less prone to developing osteoporosis, the unfavorable effects of hypogonadism on bone mass are also evident on the male gender [38]. It has been demonstrated that men with constitutional delayed puberty have a decrease in spinal and forearm BMD [39]. The hypogonadism induced by the administration of gonadotropin-releasing hormone (GnRH) leads to high-turnover bone loss [40,41]. In addition, men with isolated hypogonadotropic hypogonadism also present a decline in BMD [42]. Similarly to what is observed in patients with other causes of hypogonadism, hyperprolactinemia-induced hypogonadism has also been demonstrated to reduce BMD in men [11,13,17]. Moreover, in men with hyperprolactinemia, the reversal of hypogonadism has been associated with BMD improvement independently of the control of hyperprolactinemia [16].

Some drugs can induce hypogonadism through the development of hyperprolactinemia. PRL-raising antipsychotic agents have been appointed as the major cause of pharmacological hyperprolactinemia [20,43]. Most antipsychotic agents antagonize the actions of endogenous dopamine at the dopamine receptors type 2 (DA-2) in the brain, consequently blocking the inhibitory effect of dopamine on PRL release at the lactotrophs [44,45].

Amenorrhea or other menstrual abnormalities have long been recognized as a common secondary effect of the hyperprolactinemia induced by antipsychotic drugs [46,47]. Additionally, bone loss has been consistently related to DA-2 antagonist potency of antipsychotic drugs [44]. Higher doses of PRL-raising antipsychotic medications have been associated with increased rates of both hyperprolactinemia and hypogonadism-induced BMD loss [44,48].

In the past, estrogens were considered the main responsible for the maintenance of women's BMD and androgens for that of men. However, recent studies successfully revealed the importance of estrogens for the male skeleton. Men with abnormalities of the estrogen receptor (ER) or aromatase deficiency present, respectively, an abnormal response to estrogen and a decreased estrogen production, which result in a failure in bone mineralization and maturation [49,50]. Thus, those abnormalities can be used as models for the demonstration of the important role of estrogen on bone acquisition in men [49,50,51,52]. Some studies have been able to establish correlations between serum estradiol concentrations and bone mass in men, opening a field for discussion on the role of estrogens on bone metabolism and especially on age-related bone loss [53,54,55,56,57]. A study developed with Brazilian men with prolactinoma has confirmed that the association between BMD and estradiol levels is also present in men with hyperprolactinemia [11].

On the other hand, androgen resistance syndrome, characterized by total or partial absence of response to androgens, also results in BMD reduction [58]. In the elderly, low serum testosterone and elevated serum sex hormones-binding globulin (SHBG) levels have been associated with increased risk for osteoporosis in men [56]. Androgens have been linked with female bone metabolism as well. In premenopausal women, bone loss has been related with lower androgen levels [22]. The effects of androgens on bone physiology are both direct through the control of remodeling cycles and indirect through the transformation into estrogens [59]. In women with hyperprolactinemia, androgen levels have been directly correlated with BMD [9].

Some authors have analyzed the effects of bioavailable fractions of estrogens and androgens upon BMD. Although total estrogen and androgen levels suffer little modification throughout lifespan, serum SHBG levels increase in the elderly, which may result in a reduction of 50 to 70% of bioavailable estrogen and androgen in men [53,54,60]. Low levels of bioavailable estradiol are correlated with an increase in bone turnover and consequent bone loss, which suggests that there may be an estrogen threshold necessary for bone metabolism maintenance [22,54].

Increased levels of C-terminal telopeptide of type I collagen (CTx) have been found in patients with pharmacologically-induced hyperprolactinemia [61]. CTx is considered a marker of bone resorption and the elevation of CTx levels is compatible with the increased resorption rate secondary to the absence or decrease of sex hormones.

The bone tissue expresses estrogen and androgen receptors (ER and AR, respectively) [62]. Osteoclasts present higher concentrations of ER-alpha, while ER-beta predominate at the osteoblasts [62]. Binding to the appropriate receptors, estrogens and androgens can reduce osteoclast bone resorption and increase osteoblast collagen synthesis [62]. In hypogonadism, osteoclasts lifespan is prolonged, while the contrary happens with osteoblasts, which contributes to the deregulation of the dynamics of bone formation and resorption [63]. Estrogens and androgens are capable of decreasing the number of bone remodeling cycles by attenuating the birth rate of osteoclasts and osteoblasts from their progenitors [59]. These effects are partially due to the transcriptional regulation of genes responsible for osteoclastogenesis and mesenchymal cell replication and/or differentiation[59]. Additionally, estradiol has been shown to inhibit osteoblast and osteoclast apoptosis [63]. The osteoprotective effect of estrogen is predominantly mediated by the control of number and activity of osteoclasts [64], through the modulation of the production and activation of growth factors, such as the transforming growth factor-beta (TGF-beta) [65] and the insulin-like growth factor (IGF-1) [21], and inhibition of the synthesis of cytokines such as interleukin-6 (IL-6) [66,67].

ER have been identified on osteoblasts, osteoclasts, and osteocytes. Furthermore, AR are present on chondrocytes, osteoblasts, osteocytes, and bone marrow endothelial cells [68]. However, AR are mainly expressed on osteoblasts [59]. Androgens exert an anti-apoptotic effect on osteoblasts and osteocytes [63] and also stimulate osteoblast proliferation and differentiation, besides reducing osteoclast reabsorptive activity [69,70]. Interestingly, either ER-alpha, ER-beta or AR can transmit anti-apoptotic signals with similar efficiency, irrespective of whether the ligand is estrogen or androgen [59,63].

Steroid may also be produced *in loco* by the bone. A number of enzymes involved in the steroid synthesis are present in osteoblasts [64]. An example of local enzymatic activity is that of the 5 alpha-reductase, responsible for the conversion of testosterone to dihydrotestosterone (DHT). *Issa et al* (2002) [71] have suggested that DHT may contribute to bone metabolism through the stimulation of local AR.

Zadrosna-Sliwka et al. (2008) [72] detected an association between the cyclase activating (CAP) and cyclase inhibiting (CIP) fractions of parathormone (PTH) and estradiol levels in patients with prolactinoma, which could be ascribed to the anabolic action of both these hormone fractions on bone [73]. It is interesting to mention that a CAP/CIP ratio above 1.0 is suggestive of increased bone turnover [74].

Direct Effect of Prolactin

Some studies have shown that BMD of amenorrheic women with normal serum levels of PRL is higher than that of amenorrheic women with pathological hyperprolactinemia due to prolactinoma, suggesting that PRL could have a direct effect on bone mass independently of the influence of hypogonadism [7,75]. Moreover, correlations have been established between bone mass and the duration of hyperprolactinemia and also between BMD and serum PRL levels [13,17,76]. The direct influence of hyperprolactinemia on bone loss has been studied in men as well. Mazziotti et al. (2011) [77] correlated the prevalence of vertebral fractures in a group of men with prolactinoma solely to the duration of hyperprolactinemia. In this study, no influence of hypogonadism was detected.

Similarly to what has been observed in patients with pathological hyperprolactinemia, BMD has been inversely associated with serum PRL levels in women with pharmacologically-induced hyperprolactinemia [78]. Pharmacological hyperprolactinemia has also been linked to a decrease in BMD in adolescent boys, despite the presence of a physiological pubertal elevation on testosterone levels [79], which reinforces the importance of hyperprolactinemia as a hypogonadism-independent factor in the pathogenesis of bone loss.

Studies developed with animal models have identified PRL receptors on the osteoblasts but not on the osteoclasts [80]. Charoenphandhu et al. (2008) [81] suggested that high concentrations of PRL (1000 ng/mL) might down-regulate the expression of genes that are essential for osteoblast differentiation and function, thus contributing to the pathogenesis of bone loss. These authors demonstrated that, when osteoblasts were exposed to high concentrations of PRL, there were decreases in messenger ribonucleic acid (mRNA) expression of Runt-related transcription factor *2* (RUNX2), osteoprotegerin (OPG), and receptor activator of nuclear factor kB ligand (RANKL) of 60.49%, 72.74%, and 87.51%, respectively.

It has been established that PRL has adverse effects on the osteoblast function, leading to a decrease in bone formation in rats [82]. In these rodents, PRL exerts different effects depending on the reproductive period. While having no effect on femoral BMD and bone mineral content during pregnancy, PRL has been appointed as responsible for bone gain in early and mid-lactating periods and induced bone loss during the late lactating period [83].

In the 1980s, another mechanism was proposed in order to account for the effects of hyperprolactinemia on bone metabolism. In rats, PRL has been demonstrated to stimulate both intestinal calcium transportation and its urinary excretion [84,85]. It has been suggested that PRL is capable of stimulating the transcription of the vitamin D receptor [21]. Unfortunately, the literature offers conflicting data on the interactions between PRL and vitamin D in humans [20,35,36,85,86,87].

Parathormone-related peptide (PTHrP) presents partial homology with the PTH molecule. During the lactating period, the mammary gland is the probable source of the circulating PTHrP, which exerts a temporary modulation of calcium metabolism in face of low levels of estradiol [88]. During this period, there is an association between the serum levels of PRL and PTHrP [89]. Interestingly, PTHrP levels are elevated in 60% of men with prolactinoma-induced hyperprolactinemia and are negatively correlated with BMD in these patients [88]. Stiegler et al. (1995) [88] showed that prolactinomas presented a high immunoreactivity for PTHrP and suggested that this hormone could contribute substantially to bone loss in hyperprolactinemia.

Basal levels of calcitonin are slightly elevated in women with hyperprolactinemia, but this hormone does not seem to be responsible for bone loss in these patients, since treatment with dopamine agonists has been shown to result in BMD elevation without any effect on calcitonin levels [90].

Since IGF-1 is known to have anabolic effects on the skeleton, Torring et al. (1993)[90] studied IGF-1 concentrations in hyperprolactinemic women. However, the authors failed to find any differences between these patients and a control group. As a result, the study indicated that the inhibition of IGF-1 was not likely to be the cause of bone loss in women with hyperprolactinemia.

Bone Loss in Hyperprolactinemia

Hyperprolactinemia is considered a risk factor for the development of osteoporosis [91]. It has been demonstrated that bone resorption markers are increased and bone formation markers decreased even in hyperprolactinemic patients who present normal BMD [13]. These findings suggest that a longer disease progression would increase the risk of bone loss in these patients and eventually every patient with hyperprolactinemia could end up presenting bone loss [13,17].

The persistent increase in serum PRL levels has been associated with reduction of BMD involving both trabecular and cortical bone [8,11,17,35,92]. The former type of bone is the most seriously affect in hyperprolactinemia [7,12,13,36,93], which can be credited to the difference in turnover between trabecular and cortical bones [7,92]. Trabecular bone turnover is especially influenced by sex steroids [93]. (The importance of hypogonadism in the pathophysiology of bone loss in hyperprolactinemia was discussed in the previous section in this chapter.)

Another important feature of hyperprolactinemia-induced bone loss is its progressive nature. Thus, although the trabecular bone is the first to be involved in the pathophysiology of bone loss, progressive cortical bone loss has also been demonstrated [7,15]. However, adequate treatment of hyperprolactinemia and hypogonadism can interrupt this pattern of evolution [17].

The magnitude of bone loss in hyperprolactinemia has been associated with the duration of hypogonadism [6,15,17,92]. The restoration of menses, in women, and of normal levels of testosterone, in men, is associated with the amelioration of BMD, independently of the normalization of PRL levels [15,16,37,38]. The influence of hypogonadism is reinforced by data such as those from Biller et al. (1992) [15] who concluded that menstrual status is the most important predictor of progressive spinal osteopenia. Nevertheless, although the majority of the available data are in favor of a pivotal influence of hypogonadism on bone density of patients with hyperprolactinemia, the restoration of gonadal function has not been associated with complete normalization of bone mass and markers of bone resorption in all the studies [13,15,17,31].

On the other hand, the actual contribution of the normalization of PRL levels to the reversal of bone loss is not a unanimous finding in the literature. However, some studies detected correlations between PRL levels or the duration of hyperprolactinemia and BMD [13,17,90]. Moreover, many studies have succeeded in demonstrating that the normalization of PRL levels is able to interrupt the process of bone loss [7,8,13,14,16,31,90,94]. Nonetheless, the mere normalization of PRL levels has been considered insufficient to completely restore bone density in patients with hyperprolactinemia [13,31].

Some groups are especially prone to the deleterious effects of hyperprolactinemia and hypogonadism. In children and adolescents, hyperprolactinemia-induced bone loss is more severe than in adults [13,17,95]. The importance of the age of onset of hyperprolactinemia and its consequent hypogonadism relies on the fact that approximately 90% of peak bone mass is acquired at age eighteen [96]. Consequently, the persistently elevated levels of PRL and the consequent hypogonadism can restrict the acquisition of peak bone mass during adolescence. Additionally, a 10% increase in peak bone mass is predicted to delay the development of osteoporosis by thirteen years, suggesting that peak bone mass is the single most important determinant of the development of osteoporosis [96]. Although the treatment of hyperprolactinemia can contribute to the increase in bone density [95], the mere control of PRL levels has been proven insufficient to completely restore bone mass [17], leaving these patients with an increased risk of fracture of 2 to 3 times for each SD decrease in BMD [97].

A recent study evaluated the prevalence of vertebral fractures in men with prolactinoma and detected an index of 37.5% [77]. As expected, fractured patients had lower BMD and longer disease duration. However, no difference in fracture prevalence was identified when eugonadal and hypogonadal patients were compared [77].

An interesting finding of some of the studies on bone loss in hyperprolactinemia is that of an individual variability in BMD [15]. Although the control of hyperprolactinemia and/or secondary hypogonadism tends to partially restore BMD, some patients exhibit no change on BMD or even persistence of bone loss [13,15,17]. This variability has been observed both in trabecular and cortical bone [14,15].

CONCLUSION

Bone loss is another important and frequent complication of hyperprolactinemia. BMD should be evaluated in patients with hyperprolactinemia, with especial attention to patients with prolactinomas, pharmacologically-induced hyperprolactinemia, children, and adolescents.

The presence of low BMD is an important indication for treatment of hyperprolactinemia and secondary hypogonadism.

REFERENCES

[1] Sinha, YN; Gilligan, TA; Lee, DW; Hollinsworth, D; Markoff, E. Cleaved prolactin: Evidence for its occurrence in human pituitary gland and plasma. *J Clin Endocrinol Metab.* 1985; 60:239-243.

[2] Gillam, MP; Molitch, ME; Lombardi, G; Colao, A. Advances in the treatment of prolactinomas. *Endocr Rev.* 2006; 27 ':485-534.

[3] Faglia, G. Prolactinomas and hyperprolactinemic syndrome. In: Leslie Degroot, J Larry Jameson, ed. *Endocrinology.* Philadelphia, USA: W. B. Saunders Company; 2001:329-342.

[4] Mah, P; Webster, J. Hyperprolactinemia: Etiology, diagnosis, and management. *Semin Reprod Med.* 2002; 20:365-374.

[5] Colao, A; Di Sarno, A; Cappabianca, P et al. Gender differences in the prevalence, clinical features and response to cabergoline in hyperprolactinemia. *Eur J Endocrinol.* 2003; 148:325-331.

[6] Kayath, MJ; Lengyel, AMJ; Vieira, JGH. Prevalence and magnitude of osteopenia in patients with prolactinoma. *Brazilian J Med Biol Res.* 1993; 1993:933-941.

[7] Schlechte, J; El-Khoury, G; Kathol, M; Walkner, L. Forearm and vertebral bone mineral in treated and untreated hyperprolactinemic amenorrhea. *J Clin Endocrinol Metab.* 1987; 64:1021-1026.

[8] Greenspan, SL; Neer, RM; Ridgway, EC; Klibanski, A. Osteoporosis in men with hyperprolactinemic hypogonadism. *Ann Intern Med.* 1986; 104:777-782.

[9] Bolanowski, M; Zadrozna-Sliwka, B; Jawiarczyk, A; Syrycka, J. The influence of other than prolactin hormones on bone mineral density in women with hyperprolactinaemia of various origins. *Gynecol Endocrinol.* 2010; 26:623-627.

[10] Bussade, I; Naliato, ECO; Mendonça, LM et al. Redução da densidade mineral óssea em mulheres na menacme com prolactinoma. *Arq Bras Endcocrinol Metab.* 2007; 51:1522-1527.

[11] Naliato, ECO; Farias, MLF; Braucks, GR; Costa, FSR; Zylberberg, D; Violante, AHD. Prevalence of osteopenia in men with prolactinoma. *J Endocrinol Invest.* 2005; 28:12-17.

[12] Naliato, ECO; Violante, AHD; Caldas, D et al. Bone density in women with prolactinoma treated with dopamine agonists. *Pituitary.* 2008; 11:21-28.

[13] Di Somma, C; Colao, A; Di Sarno, A et al. Bone marker and bone density responses to dopamine agonist therapy in hyperprolactinemic males. *J Clin Endocrinol Metab.* 1998; 83:807-813.

[14] Klibanski, A; Greenspan, S. Increase in bone mass after treatment of hyperprolactinemic amenorrhea. *N Engl J Med.* 1986; 315:542-546.

[15] Biller, BMK; Baum, HB; Rosenthal, DI; Saxe, VC; Charpie, PM; Klibanski, A. Progressive trabecular osteopenia in women with hyperprolactinemia amenorrhea. *J Clin Endocrinol Metab.* 1992; 75:692-697.

[16] Greenspan, SL; Oppenheim, D; Klibanski, A. Importance of gonadal steroids to bone mass in men with hyperprolactinemic hypogonadism. *Ann Intern Med.* 1989; 110:526-531.

[17] Colao, A; Di Somma, C; Loche, S et al. Prolactinomas in adolescents: persistent bone loss after 2 years of prolactin normalization. *Clin Endocrinol.* 2000; 52:319-327.

[18] Drinkwater, BL; Nilson, K; Ott, SM; Chesnut III, CH. Menstrual history as a determinant of current bone density in young athletes. *JAMA.* 1990; 263:545-548.

[19] Santoro, N. Update in hyper- and hypogonadotropic amenorrhea. *J Clin Endocrinol Metab.* 2011; 96:3281–3288.

[20] Kishimoto, T; Watanabe, K; Shimada, N; Makita, K; Yagi, G; Kashima, H. Antipsychotic-induced hyperprolactinemia inhibits the hypothalamo-pituitary-gonadal axis and reduces bone mineral density in male patients with schizophrenia. *J Clin Psychiatry.* 2008; 69:385-391.

[21] Meczekalski, B; Podfigurna-Stopa, A; Genazzani, AR. Hypoestrogenism in young women and its influence on bone mass density. *Gyncol Endocrinol.* 2010; 26:652-657.

[22] Slemenda, C; Longcope, C; Peacock, M; Hui, S; Johnston, CC. Sex steroids, bone mass, and bone loss. *J Clin Invest.* 1996; 97:14-21.

[23] Hui, SL; Perkins, AJ; Zhou, L et al. Bone loss at the femoral neck in premenopausal white women: Effects of weight change and sex-hormone levels. *J Clin Endocrinol Metab.* 2002; 87:1539-1543.

[24] Riggs, BLKS; Melton III, J. Sex steroids and the construction and conservation of the adult skeleton. *Endocr Rv.* 2002; 23:279-302.

[25] Magrini, G; Ebner, JR; Burckhardt, P; Felber, JP. Study on the relationship between plasma prolactin levels and androgen metabolism in men. *J Clin Endocrinol Metab.* 1976; 43:944-947.

[26] Kauppila, A; Leinonen, P; Vihko, R; Ylöstalo, P. Metoclopramide-induced hyperprolactinemia impairs ovarian follicle maturation and

corpus luteum function in women. *J Clin Endocrinol Metab.* 1982; 54:955-960.
[27] Bouchard, P; Lagoguey, M; Brailly, S; Schaison, G. Gonadotropin-Releasing Hormone pulsatile administration restores luteinizing hormone pulsatility and normal testosterone levels in males with hyperprolactinemia. *J Clin Endocrinol Metab.* 1985; 60:258-262.
[28] Carter, JN; Tyson, JE; Tollis, G; Van Vliet, S; Fairman, C; Friesen, HG. Prolactin secreting tumors and hypogonadism in 22 men. *N Engl J Med.* 1978; 299:847-852.
[29] Pinzone, JJ; Katznelson, L; Danila, DC; Pauler, DK; Miller, CS; Klibanski, A. Primary medical therapy of micro- and macroprolactinomas in men. *J Clin Endocrinol Metab.* 2000; 85:3053-3057.
[30] Braucks, GR; Naliato, ECO; Tabet, ALO; Gadelha, MR; Violante, AHD. Aspectos clínicos e terapêuticos de prolactinomas em homens. *Arq Neuropsiquiatr.* 2003; 61:1004-1010.
[31] Schlechte, J; Walkner, L; Kathol, M. A longitudinal analysis of premenopausal bone loss in healthy women and women with hyperprolactinemia. *J Clin Endocrinol Metab.* 1992; 75:698-703.
[32] Adler, RA; Evani, R; Mansouri, A; Krieg Jr, RJ. Relative effects of prolactin excess and estrogen deficiency on bone in rats. 1998; 47:425-428.
[33] Nystrom, E; Leman, J; Lundberg, PA et al. Bone mineral content in normally menstruating women with hyperpolactenaemia. *Horm Res.* 1988; 29:214-217.
[34] Ciccarelli, E; Savino, L; Carlevatto, V, Bertagna, A; Isaia, GC; Camanni, F. Vertebral bone density in non-amenorrhoeic hyperprolactinemia. *Clin Endocrinol.* 1988; 28:1-6.
[35] Klibanski, A; Neer, RM; Beitins, IZ; Ridgway, EC; Zervas, NT; McArthur, JW. Decreased bone density in hyperprolactinemic women. *N Engl J Med.* 1980; 303:1511-1514.
[36] Koppelman, MCS; Kurtz, DW; Morrish, K et al. Vertebral bone mineral content in hyperprolactinemic women. *J Clin Endocrinol Metab.* 1984; 59:1050-1053.
[37] Klibanski, A; Biller, BMK; Rosenthal, DI; Schoenfeld, DA; Saxe, V. Effects of prolactin and estrogen deficiency in amenorrheic bone loss. *J Clin Endocrinol Metab.* 1988; 67:124-130.

[38] Jackson, JA; Kleerekoper, M; Parfitt, AM. Symptomatic osteoporosis in a man with hyperprolactinemic hypogonadism. *Ann Intern Med.* 1986; 105:543-545.
[39] Finkelstein, J; Klibanski, A; Nerr, R. A longitudinal evaluation of bone mineral density in adult men histories of delay puberty. *J Clin Endocrinol Metab.* 1996; 81:1152-1155.
[40] Mittan, D; Lee, S; Miller, E; Perez, RC; Basler, JW; Bruder, JM. Bone loss following hypogonadism in men with prostate cancer treated with GnRH analogs. *J Clin Endocrinol Metab.* 2002; 87:3656-3661.
[41] Goldray, D; Weisman, Y; Jaccard, N; Merdler, C; Chen, J; Matzkin, H. Decreased bone density in elderly men treated with the gonadotropin-releasing hormone agonist decapeptyl (D-Trp-GnRH). *J Clin Endocrinol Metab.* 1993; 76:288-290.
[42] Guo, C; Jones, T; Eastell, R. Treatment of isolated hypogonadotropic hypogonadism effect on bone mineral density & bone turnover. *J Clin Endocrinol Metab.* 1997; 82:658-665.
[43] Petty, RG. Prolactin and antipsychotic medications: Mechanism of action. *Schizophr Res.* 1999; 35:S67-S73.
[44] O'Keane, V. Antipsychotic-induced hyperprolactinaemia, hypogonadism and osteoporosis in the treatment of schizophrenia. *J Psychopharmacol.* 2008; 22:70-75.
[45] Rosenbloom, AL. Hyperprolactinemia with Antipsychotic Drugs in Children and Adolescents. *Int J Pediatr Endocrinol.* 2010; 2010.
[46] 46 Beumont, PJ; Gelder, MG; Friesen, GH et al. The effects of phenothiazines on endocrine function: I. Patients with inappropriate lactation and amenorrhoea. *Br J Psychiatry.* 1974; 124:413-419.
[47] Mancini, AM; Guitelman, A; Vargas, CA; Debeljuk, L; Aparicio, NJ. Effect of sulpiride on serum prolactin levels in humans. *J Clin Endocrinol Metab.* 1976; 42:181-184.
[48] Meaney, AM; Smith, S; Howes, OD; O'Brien, M; Murray, RM; O'Keane, V. Effects of long-term prolactin-raising antipsychotic medication on bonemineral density in patients with schizophrenia. *Br J Psychiatry.* 2004; 184:503-508.
[49] Morishima, A; Grumbach, MM; Simpson, ER; Fisher, C; Qin, K. Aromatase deficiency in male and female siblings caused by a novel mutation and the physiological role of estrogens. *J Clin Endocrinol Metab.* 1995; 80:3689-3698.
[50] Lorentzon, M; Lorentzon, R; Bäckström, T; Nordström, P. Estrogen receptor gene polymorphism, but not estradiol levels is related to bone

density in healthy adolescent boys: a cross-sectional and longitudinal study. *J Clin Endocrinol Metab.* 1999; 84:4597-4601.

[51] Byers, RJ; Hoyland, JA; Braidman, IP. Osteoporosis in men: a cellular endocrine perspective of an increasingly common clinical problem. *J Endocrinol.* 2001; 168:353-362.

[52] Herrmann, BL; Saller, B; Janssen, O et al. Impact of estrogen replacement therapy in a male with congenital aromatase deficiency caused by a novel mutation in the CYP19 gene. *J Clin Endocrinol Metab.* 2002; 87:5476-5484.

[53] Khosla, S; Melton III, J; Atlinson, EJ; O'Fallon, WM; Klee, GG; Riggs, L. Relationship of serum sex steroid levels and bone turnover markers with bone mineral density in men and women: A key role for bioavailable estrogen. *J Clin Endocrinol Metab.* 1998; 83:2266-2274.

[54] Khosla, S; Melton III, LJ; Atkinson, EJ; O'Fallon, WM. Relationship of serum sex steroid levels to longitudinal changes in bone density in young versus elderly men. *J Clin Endocrinol Metab.* 2001; 86:3555-3561.

[55] Ongphiphadhanakul, B; Rajatanavin, R; Chanprasertyothin, S; Piaseu, N; Chailurkit, L. Serum oestradiol and oestrogen-receptor gene polymorphism are associated with bone mineral density independently of serum testosterone in normal males. *Clin Endocrinol.* 1998; 49:803-809.

[56] Center, JR; Nguyen, TV; Sambrook, PN; Eisman, JA. Hormonal and biochemical parameters in the determination of osteoporosis in elderly men. *J Clin Endocrinol Metab.* 1999; 84:3626-3635.

[57] Barrett-Connor, E; Mueller, JE; von Mühlen, DG; Laughlin, GA; Schneider, DL; Sartoris, DJ. Low levels of estradiol are associated with vertebral fractures in older men, but not in women: the Rancho Bernardo Study. *J Clin Endocrinol Metab.* 2000; 85:219-223.

[58] Marcus, R; Leary, D; Schneider, DL; Shane, E; Favus, M; Quigley, CA. The contribution of testosterone to skeletal development and maintenance: lessons from the androgen insensitivity syndrome. *J Clin Endocrinol Metab.* 2000; 85:1032-1037.

[59] Balasch, J. Sex steroids and bone: current perspectives. *Hum Reprod Update.* 2003; 9:207-222.

[60] Lopes, RF; Ferreira, AGJ; Coeli, CM; Farias, MLF. Low body mass index and declining sex steroids explain most age-related bone loss in Brazilian men. *Osteoporos Int.* 2009; 20:1175- 1182.

[61] Doknic, M; Maric, NP; Britvic, D et al. Bone remodeling, bone mass and weight gain in patients with stabilized schizophrenia in real-life conditions treated with long-acting injectable risperidone. *Neuroendocrinology.* 2011; 94:246-254.

[62] Zhang-Wong, JH; Seeman, MV. Antipsychotic drugs, menstrual regularity and osteoporosis risk. *Arch Womens Ment Health.* 2002; 5:93-98.

[63] Manolagas, S. Birth and death of bone cells: Basic regulatory mechanisms and implications for the pathogenesis and treatment of osteoporosis. *Endocr Rev.* 2000; 21:115-137.

[64] Compston, J. Sex steroids and bone. *Physiological Rev.* 2001; 81:419-447.

[65] Robinson, JA; Riggs, BL; Spelsberg, TC; Oursler, MJ. Osteoclasts and transforming growth factor-ß: estrogen-mediated isoform-specific regulation of production. *Endocrinology.* 1996; 137:615-621.

[66] Girasole, G; Jilka, RL; Passeri, G et al. 17beta-estradiol inhibits interleukin-6 production by bone marrow-derived cells and osteoblasts in vitro: a potential mechanism for the antiosteoporotic effect of estrogens. *J Clin Invest.* 1992; 89:883-891.

[67] Srivastava, S; Weitzmann, MN; Kimble, RB et al. Estrogen blocks M-CSF gene expression and osteoclast formation by regulating phosphorylation of Egr-1 and its interaction with Sp-1. *J Clin Invest.* 1998; 102:1850-1859.

[68] Abu, EO; Horner, A; Kusec, V; Triffitt, JT; Compston, JE. The localization of androgen receptors in human bone. *J Clin Endocrinol Metab.* 1997; 82:3493-3497.

[69] Kasperk, CH; Wakley, GK; Hierl, T; Ziegler, R. Gonadal and adrenal androgens are potent regulators of human bone metabolism in vitro. *J Bone Miner Res.* 1997; 12:464-471.

[70] Pederson, L; Kremer, M; Judd, J et al. Androgens regulate bone resorption activity of isolated osteoclasts in vitro. *Proc Natl Acad Sci.* 1999; 96:505-510.

[71] Issa, S; Schnabel D; Feix, M et al. Human osteoblast-like cells express predominantly steroid 5alpha-reductase type 1. *J Clin Endocrinol Metab.* 2002; 87:5401-5407.

[72] Zadrozna-Sliwka, B; Bolanowski, M; Jawiarczyk, A; Kaluzny, M; Syrycka, J. The role of cyclase activating (CAP) and cyclase inhibiting (CIP) parathormone fractions in the assessment of bone metabolism

disturbances in women with hyperprolactinemia of various origin. *Neuro Endocrinol Lett.* 2008; 29:178-184.
[73] Franek, E; Piwowarska, I; Bulanowski, M; Kokot, F; Wiecek, A. Serum concentration of 1-84 (cyclase-activating) and 7-84 (cyclase-inhibiting) parathormone in elderly women with low mineral density of the trabecular bone. *Endokrynol Pol.* 2008; 59:471–476.
[74] Kameda, T; Mano, H; Yuasa, T et al. Estrogen inhibits bone resorption by directly inducing apoptosis of the bone-resorbing osteoclasts. *J Exp Med.* 1997; 186:489–495.
[75] Schlechte, J; Sherman, B; Martin, R. Bone density in amenorrheic women with and without hyperprolactinemia. *J Clin Endocrinol Metab.* 1983; 56:1120-1123.
[76] Greenspan, S; Oppenheim, D; Klibanski, A. Importance of gonadal steroids to bone mass in men with hyperprolactinemic hypogonadism. *Ann Intern Med.* 1986; 110:526-531.
[77] Mazziotti, G; Porcelli, T; Mormando, M et al. Vertebral fractures in males with prolactinoma. *Endocrine.* 2011; 39:288-293.
[78] Liu-Seifert, H; Kinon, BJ; Ahl, J; Lamberson, S. Osteopenia associated with increased prolactin and aging in psychiatric patients treated with prolactin-elevating antipsychotics. *Ann N Y Acad Sci.* 2004; 1032:297-298.
[79] Calarge, CA; Zimmerman, B; Xie, D; Kuperman, S; Schlechte, JA. A cross-sectional evaluation of the effect of risperidone and selective serotonin reuptake inhibitors on bone mineral density in boys. *J Clin Psychiatry.* 2010; 71:338-347.
[80] Clément-Lacroix, P; Damotte, D; Goffin, V et al. Osteoblasts are a new target for prolactin: analysis of bone formation in prolactin receptor knockout mice. *J Clin Endocrinol Metab.* 1999; 140:96-105.
[81] Charoenphandhu, N; Teerapornpuntakit, J; Methawasin, M; Wongdee, K; Thongchote, K; Krishnamra, N. Prolactin decreases expression of Runx2, osteoprotegerin, and RANKL in primary osteoblasts derived from tibiae of adult female rats. *Can J Physiol Pharmacol.* 2008; 86:240-248.
[82] Coss, D; Yang, L; Kuo, CB; Xu, X; Luben, RA; Walker, AM. Effects of prolactin on osteoblast alkaline phosphatase and bone formation in the developing rat. *Am J Physiol.* 2000; 279:E1216-E1225.
[83] Suntornsaratoon, P; Wongdee, K; Krishnamra, N; Charoenphandhu, N. Femoral bone mineral density and bone mineral content in

bromocriptine-treated pregnant and lactating rats. *J Physiol Sci.* 2010; 60:1-8.

[84] Pahuja, D; Deluca, H. Stimulation of intestinal calcium transport and bone calcium mobilization by prolactin in vitamin D-deficient rats. *Science.* 1981; 214:1038-1039.

[85] Kumar, R; Abboud, C; Riggs, B. The effect of elevated prolactin levels on plasma 1,25-dihydroxyvitamin D and intestinal absorption of calcium. *Mayo Clin Proc.* 1980; 55:51-53.

[86] Adams, ND; Garthwaite, TL; Gray, RW; Hagen, TC; Lemann Jr, J. The interrelations among prolactin 1,25-dihydrovitamin D, and parathyroid hormone in humans. *J Clin Endocrinol Metab.* 1979; 49:628-630.

[87] Brown, D; Spanos, E; Macintire, I. Role of pituitary hormones in regulating renal vitamin D metabolism in man. *Br Med J.* 1980; 1:277-278.

[88] Stiegler, C; Leb, G; Kleinert, R et al. Plasma levels of parathyroid hormone-related peptide are elevated in hyperprolactinemia and correlated to bone density status. *J Bone Miner Res.* 1995; 10:751-759.

[89] Kovacs, C. Calcium and bone metabolism in pregnancy and lactation. *J Clin Endocrinol Metab.* 2001; 86:2344-2648.

[90] Tørring, O; Isberg, B; Sjöberg, HE; Bucht, E; Hulting, AL. Plasma calcitonin, IGF-I levels and vertebral bone mineral density in hyperprolactinemic women during bromocriptine treatment. *Acta Endocrinol (Copenh).* 1993; 128:423-427.

[91] Vartej, P; Poiana, C; Vartej, I. Effects of hyperprolactinemia on osteoporotic fracture risk in premenopausal women. *Gynecol Endocrinol.* 2001; 15:43-47.

[92] Seeman, E; Melton III, L; O'Fallon, WM; Riggs, BL. Risk factors for spinal osteoporosis in men. *Am J Med.* 1983; 75:977-983.

[93] Cann, CE; Martin, MC; Genant, HK; Jaffe, RB. Decreased spinal mineral content in amenorrheic women. *JAMA.* 1984; 251:626-630.

[94] Caraceni, MP; Corghi, E; Ortolani, S; Casazza, S; D'Alberton, A; Motta, T. Increased forearm bone mineral content after bromocriptine treatment in hyperprolactinemia. *Calcif Tissue Int.* 1985; 37:687-689.

[95] Galli-Tsinopoulou, A; Nousia-Arvanitakis, S; Mitsiakos, G; Karamouzis, M; Dimitriadis, A. Osteopenia in children and adolescents with hyperprolactinemia. *J Pediatr Endocrinol Metab.* 2000; 13:439-441.

[96] Hernandez, CJ; Beaupré, GS; Carter, DR. A theoretical analysis of the relative influences of peak BMD, age-related bone loss and menopause on the development of osteoporosis. *Osteoporos Int.* 2003; 14:843–847.
[97] Matkovic, V. Skeletal development & bone turnover revisited. *J Clin Endocrinol Metab.* 1996; 81:2013-2016.

In: Bone Loss
Editor: Kuo-Cheng Lu
ISBN: 978-1-62417-169-7

Chapter 6

THE ROLE OF MICROBIAL, GENETIC AND MODIFYING (COMORBIDITIES) FACTORS IN THE INFLAMMATORY BONE LOSS ASSOCIATED TO PERIODONTITIS

Gustavo Pompermaier Garlet[1], Marcela Claudino[2], Carolina Favaro Francisconi[1], Ana Claudia de Araujo Pires[1], Celso Martins Queiroz-Junior[3], Tarcília Aparecida da Silva[3], Gerson Francisco de Assis[1], Ana Paula Campanelli[1] and Ana Paula Favaro Trombone[4]

[1]Department of Biological Sciences, School of Dentistry of Bauru, São Paulo University - FOB/USP

[2]Instituto Latino Americano de Pesquisa e Ensino Odontológico - ILAPEO

[3]Department of Oral Pathology, Faculty of Dentistry, Universidade Federal de Minas Gerais – UFMG

[4]Pathology Division, Instituto Lauro de Souza Lima – ILSL, Brazil

ABSTRACT

The development of regulated immune responses is essential in the balance between tolerance and immunity to antigens. Immune-related disorders are the result of inappropriate destruction of normal tissue by unbalanced immune inflammatory reactions, and comprise autoimmune (a failure of immune self-tolerance) and inflammatory disorders (an excessive inflammatory reaction to exogenous antigens). Among highly prevalent chronic inflammatory diseases, periodontal diseases (PD) are characterized by the inflammatory bone resorption of the teeth supporting structures. PD is the most prevalent form of bone pathology in humans and a modifying factor of the systemic health of patients. PD presents a complex etiology, where microbial factors trigger a chronic inflammatory immune response, whose nature and strength are related to the lesions stability or progression. Such response, and consequently the PD outcome, also can be modulated by local, systemic and environmental factors, and by the host genetic background, but the extent of each contributing factor to the pathogenesis of PD remains unknown. In fact, over the years the contribution of microbial, genetic and modifying factors (a series of co-morbidities including diabetes and rheumatoid arthritis) have been investigated in PD. However, in the view of the potential overlapping or additive/synergistic effects of such factors in alveolar bone loss, its individual investigation does not allow the determination of its individual and exact role in the determination of bone loss severity that typify PD. Therefore, this review article will discuss the individual and associated risks that single nucletotide polymorphisms (SNPs), classic pathogens (such as the red complex and *A. actinomycetemcomitans*) and modifying factors (such as diabetes and rheumatoid arthritis) confer to the PD-associated bone loss. Interestingly, the genetic-environmental interaction is quite diverse, ranging from additive effects to dominant scenarios, where genetic predisposition and the intensity and frequency of microbial challenge can result in distinct outcomes. Also, the modulator effect of co-morbidities is characterized beyond a simple exacerbation of inflammatory reaction and bone loss process, comprising a significant modulation of host responsiveness, which even involves the participation of commensal flora.

INTRODUCTION

Periodontal diseases (PDs) are highly prevalent chronic infectious inflammatory diseases characterized by the destruction of tooth-supporting structures, which include the irreversible resorption of alveolar bone. In epidemiologic terms, PDs comprise the most common osteolytic disease, and different PD forms are described to affect the majority of the adult population around the world, being also considered a modifying factor of the systemic health of patients [1-6]. PDs etiology basically involves microbial factors that trigger host inflammatory and immune response.

Even in oral (and periodontal) healthy conditions (i.e. in the absence of PDs), the periodontal tissues are exposed to potentially pathogenic microorganisms (from the microbial biofilm) and, to some extent, are capable to tolerate these aggressions maintaining the local tissue homeostasis. However, quantitative and qualitative changes in the microbial biofilm (e.g. when gram-negative species outnumber gram-positive bacteria) may result in increased antigenic challenge in the periodontal tissues (specifically in the gingival sulcus and junctional epithelium – for periodontal tissues structure, please consult [7]). Importantly, the lipopolyssacharide (LPS) of gram-negative bacteria are considered the main factor for triggering the initial events of host response [8-11]. In addition to the relative unspecific stimulatory effects of LPS, periodontpathogens such as *A. actinomycetemcomitans, P. gingivalis, T. denticola* and *T. forsythia*, usually associated to increased severity of periodontal disease, present several specific virulence factors, which allow not only colonization, survival and proliferation of such bacteria in oral environment; but also tissue invasion and significant modulation of host defense mechanisms [9-10, 12].

While the presence of pathogenic microorganism is essential to development of disease, the amplification and progression of this process are dependent on the nature and intensity of the response generated by the host in response to bacterial challenge [13-17]. This response involves inflammatory (mainly vascular events that will enable leukocyte migration) and immunological events; initially cellular events involved in leukocyte migration, in which adhesion molecules, chemokines and cytokines control the selective migration of different leukocyte subtypes in presence of chemotactic gradients, and subsequently the effector and regulatory stages of immune response by these distinct leukocyte subpopulations. These events result in the presence of inflammatory cells and mediators in the connective tissue underlying gingival epithelium and surrounding alveolar bone [18-20].

The nature and intensity of this response has been associated to progression or stability of periodontal lesions [13-16]. Furthermore, the host-microbial interaction, and consequently the establishment, progression and outcome of PDs, may still be influenced by local, systemic, environmental, genetic and epigenetic factors [15, 21-26]. Indeed, along the last decades all these factors have been sequentially associated with the modulation of PD, and confer to PDs a complex and multifactorial nature. However, the majority of studies focused in the mechanistic basis of PD and associated bone loss have been focused in individual factors, and how the interaction between them influences PD etiology remains an unanswered question. Also, since some of these factors are potentially overlapping, individual investigations do not provide a full picture of the actual scenario, and the putative role of each variable in the overall PDs pathogenesis context remains unknown. In this chapter, the relative role of microbial, genetic and modifying factors in the inflammatory bone loss associated to periodontitis will be discussed, considering initially the individual involvement of each factor at a glance, and in the sequence the recent progresses in the understanding of its combined role in the determination of PDs outcome.

Inflammatory Immune Response in Periodontal Environment and Its Role in Alveolar Bone Loss

The Classic Inflammatory Osteolytic Cytokines

Classic pro-inflammatory cytokines, such as TNF-α and IL-1β, have been associated with the pathogenesis of PDs. These mediators, involved in several steps of leukocyte migration process, are also characteristic inducer of proteases expression, and contribute to the differentiation and activation of osteoclasts; events directly associated to connective tissue degradation and bone resorption in periodontal environment [13-14, 18]. Relatively recent studies have been clarifying the molecular basis of soft and mineralized tissue destruction in the course of PD, and two major systems (MMPs/TIMPs and RANK/RANKL/OPG) have been associated with disease progression. Matrix metalloproteinases (MMPs) are a family of proteases capable of degrading various extracellular matrix components in several physiological and pathological processes. The activation of MMPs is regulated by a group of endogenous proteins named tissue inhibitors of metalloproteinases (TIMPs) that are capable of inhibiting almost every member of the MMP family in a non-specific way [27-28]. In physiological conditions, the TIMPs are in balance with the MMPs and the matrix is remodeled in a highly regulated pathway. However, in many disease processes, including PDs, the levels of MMPs are elevated without a concomitant increase in TIMPs, resulting in tissue destruction [28-31]. Moreover, RANK/RANKL/OPG system is also strictly involved in the pathogenesis of PDs due their role in the control of osteoclasts differentiation and activation. The engagement between RANKL (ligand of receptor activator of nuclear factor-kB) and its receptor RANK [receptor activator of nuclear factor-kB], which is expressed on osteoclastic precursors, is the major osteoclastogenic pathway. The effects of RANKL are counteracted by osteoprotegerin (OPG), a decoy RANKL receptor, which strongly inhibits bone resorption by preventing RANK–RANKL engagement [32-35]. As previously described to MMPs/TIMPS system, studies demonstrated that the balance between RANKL and OPG levels is an important factor to determinate PD activity and progression [Teng 2000, Crotti *et al.* 2003, Liu *et al.* 2003, Garlet *et al.* 2004, Mogi *et al.* 2004].

Therefore, the development of PDs involves primarily an inflammatory pathway, in which TNF-α and IL-1β (along with other inflammatory cytokines such as IL-1α and IL-6) upregulate inflammatory cells migration and expression of MMPs and RANKL, resulting in an intense catabolic activity that culminates with the alveolar bone loss and the concurrent destruction of soft periodontal tissues [13-14, 18]. Accordingly, studies in experimental models of PDs confirmed the putative role of TNF-α and IL-1β [Graves and Cochran, 2003; Cochran, 2008; Graves, 2008; Garlet, Cardoso et al., 2007]. However the inhibition of these cytokines [or their absence in genetically modified animals] results in a partial reduction in the severity of the disease, suggesting that other cytokines/molecules are also involved in the pathogenesis of PDs operating in a complex auto-regulatory network [Graves and Cochran, 2003; Cochran, 2008; Graves, 2008; Garlet, Cardoso et al., 2007]. In fact, other cytokines than TNF-α and IL-1β are described to play active roles in PD lesions.

Interleukin (IL)-10 is a potent pleiotropic cytokine with marked anti-inflammatory and immunosuppressive functions, which include a role as an important regulator of alveolar bone homeostasis in oral environment in both homeostatic and inflammatory conditions [36-38]. In the pathogenesis of bone lytic diseases such as PDs, IL-10 presents a critical role in lesions outcome [39-41]. IL-10 counteracts inflammatory bone loss through the downregulation of the signaling and activity of pro-inflammatory cytokines such as TNF-α and IL-1β. Indeed, IL-10 presents a protective role toward tissue destruction inhibiting both MMPs and RANK systems [30, 42] through the upregulation TIMPs [27, 43] and OPG [33, 39].Besides its role in the attenuation of inflammatory bone loss, IL-10 seems to have an important homeostatic role over skeletal system. It has been suggested that IL-10 promoter gene polymorphisms are associated with reduced bone mineral density and predisposition to osteoporosis development [44]. In addition, evaluating bone metabolism in IL-10 gene knockout (KO) mice, it was observed that IL-10 lack accelerates alveolar bone loss in healthy periodontal environment [37-38, 45].

At this point, it is possible to suggest that an overall balance between pro- (TNF-α and IL-1β) and anti- (IL-10) inflammatory cytokines is the central pathway in the determination of bone loss activity and PD progression. Also, in this context, it is reasonable to suggest that variations in the levels of TNF-α, IL-1β and IL-10 could account for parallel variations in the disease outcome, and interestingly, PD patients characteristically present a relatively high degree in the variation of such cytokines levels in the lesions [46-48]. Also, factors such as specific bacteria or genetic factors, that influence the expression of such cytokines, and the overall pro- versus anti-inflammatory balance, can potentially modulate PD outcome, as will be further discussed. In addition, other cytokines can participate in the local host response and greatly influence the levels of pro- versus anti-inflammatory expression, and also directly interfere in the bone loss process along PD evolution.

T Helper Cytokines

Beyond classical proinflammatory pathway previously described, mainly associated to innate immune responses, adaptive immunity derived cytokines can play important roles in the determination of inflammation-mediated osteolysis severity and consequently in the determination of PD outcome. Indeed, cytokines produced by T helper (Th) cells can actively attenuate or enhance of the pro-inflammatory response and degree of bone loss in periodontal tissues [4, 19, 49-52]. In this context, patients with aggressive periodontitis [a form of periodontal disease characterized by extensive bone loss and high disease severity] present an increased expression of IFN-γ, the prototypical cytokine of Th1- type, which correlates with higher levels of MMPs (MMP-1, 2 and 9) and RANKL [30, 53]. Conversely, patients with chronic periodontitis (characterized generally by low severity and slow progression) presents a higher expression of IL-4 (the typical Th2 cytokines) and IL-10 (also considered a Th2-type cytokine in certain circumstances) with anti-inflammatory characteristics [30, 53]. It has been demonstrated that an increased expression of these mediators was correlated with augmented expression of TIMPs and OPG, which possibly accounts for lower bone resorption and consequent reduction in periodontal disease severity [30, 46, 53]. Then, the predominance of a Th1 response seems to enhance the classical inflammatory pathway involving TNF-α and IL-1β, while high levels of Th2-type mediators seems to control (even partially) the progression of periodontal disease. However, despite the significant association between Th1 and Th2 cytokines with distinct patterns of bone loss and PD severity, the individual variations in the levels of these cytokines do not seem to fully explain the variation in lesions severity. Recently other subpopulations of lymphocytes with relevant immunoregulatory characteristics and able to produce prototypical cytokines able to modulate bone loss process were identified in PD lesions [17, 54-55].

Among the subtypes of cells with suppressor or regulatory functions, a subpopulation of CD4 T cells that co express constitutively CD25 (the alpha chain of receptor IL-2), collectively called Tregs (regulatory T cells) are described as essential for the control of immune response, preventing or attenuating the deleterious effects of exacerbated responses [56-64]. Besides constitutive expression of CD25, these cells are characterized by this phenotype: $CD5^{high}$, $GITR^{+}$, $CD38^{+}$, $CD103^{+}$, $CD45^{low}$. In addition, the expression of the transcription factor FOXP3 is unique feature of $CD4^{+}$ $CD25^{+}$ regulatory T cells, being essential to the development and function of these cells [58-62]. Although some controversies concerning to mechanisms of action, it is believed that these cells exerts its functions in a manner dependent on cell-cell contact through the inhibitory molecule CTLA4, or through the production of cytokines such as TGF-β, IL-10 and IL-35 [58-64]. Concerning to PDs, higher levels of regulatory T cells in periodontal lesions have been recently demonstrated, being related with expression of IL-10 and TGF-β. However, possible associations between regulatory T cells and control (or interferences in the control) of periodontopathogens remains poorly known [54]. Recent studies demonstrate that Treg cells can be subdivided into subpopulations, but the absence of definitive markers does not allow definitive approaches in this context. In this way, such subdivisions remain controversial in the literature. Some studies have been described that activated Treg cells leads to suppression of proliferation of other T cells, and can also block or reduce the production of inflammatory mediators by different subpopulations of leukocytes [58, 65-66].

In previous studies, the presence of Tregs cells was characterized in periodontal lesions [54]. The expression of FOXP3, CTLA4, GITR, CD45RO and CD103 was associated with production of IL-10 and TGF-beta. Concerning to experimental models, it has been demonstrated that the absence of the regulatory function of Treg cells [due by anti-GITR treatment] results in higher levels of alveolar bone resorption, accompanied by increased migration of inflammatory cells into the periodontal tissues. In fact, such phenomena are associated with an increased expression of inflammatory cytokines, RANKL and MMPs, and a lower expression of IL-10, TGF-b and CTLA4 [54, 67].

Interestingly, interactions between regulatory T cells and different microorganisms have been described. While commensal pathogens seem to induce an increased migration of regulatory T cells, some pathogens can induce the activity of regulatory T cells as evasion mechanism to overcome the host protective immune response. Indeed, the effective immunoregulatory role of regulatory T cells may be harmful, being determinant in maintaining a latent state in different infections, facilitating the survival of pathogens and allowing reactivation of the disease [58-65, 68-69].

Beyond regulatory T cells, Th17 cells, characterized by interleukin-17 [IL-17] production, have been implicated in the immunoregulation of various pathological processes [17, 70-71]. The development of Th17 cells involves activation of the transcription factor RORg stimulated by TGF-β, IL-6 and IL-21, and its polarization can be inhibited by Th1 and Th2 cytokines. Previous studies suggest the influence of Th17 cells in the pathogenesis of autoimmune inflammatory diseases such as rheumatoid arthritis [72-73], and that IL-17 plays an important role in the stimulation of osteoclastogenesis to induce expression of RANKL in patients with rheumatoid arthritis [74]. It shares certain molecular mechanisms with periapical lesions related to the process of osteolysis associated with chronic inflammation. Initial investigations regarding to the role of IL-17 in human oral diseases has been developed [54], demonstrating that the presence of this cytokine in the periodontal lesions has been correlated with expression of metalloproteinases, interleukins such as pro-inflammatory IL-1β and TNF-α [75] and the induction of bone resorption [72, 76], contributing to increased disease severity [77].

Subsequent studies confirmed the strong expression of this cytokine in chronic periapical lesions [77-78], being associated with exacerbation of inflammatory process, due stimulation of IL-8 expression. However, the relationship between IL-17 and the modulation of expression of other cytokines and osteoclastogenic factors remains poorly described. In this context, an experimental study describes the induction of chronic periapical lesions in the absence of IL-17, being results completely different from other previous studies. Therefore, a re-evaluation seems to be necessary, besides the investigation of putative mechanisms related to the modulation of periapical lesions severity by IL-17. Preliminary results from our group concerning to the analysis of cytokine profile in human periapical granulomas suggest that Th1 and Th17 pathways can positively modulate the expression of RANKL, but in an independent pathway, suggesting that such pathways may be mutually inhibitory. Interestingly, the characterization of Th17 cells has led to review of pathological mechanisms of certain diseases such as rheumatoid arthritis, which was typically considered as a result of the action of Th1 cells and their characteristic cytokine, IFN-γ, even when some events could not be fully explained in this model [17]. Recent studies have correlated the presence of IL-17 in diseased periodontal tissue to expression of IL-1β, TNF-α, MMPs and, consequently, bone resorption induction [75-76], suggesting the putative role of Th17 cells in the pathogenesis of PDs. Thus, we also demonstrated higher levels of IL-17, IL-6 and IL-23, cytokines related to Th17 response, expressed in periodontal lesions [55].

Thus, it is reasonable consider that, beyond the participation of classical inflammatory pathway mediated by IL-1β and TNF-α, and modulated by Th1, Th2 cells, Th17 and regulatory T cells are also involved in the immunoregulation of periodontal lesions [17, 21]. Therefore, as previously mentioned to the pro- versus anti-inflammatory archetype, factors that can influence the overall Th activity and balance in periodontal tissues can directly impact the bone loss activity in periodontal lesions. Among these factors, we can mention the genetic influences, specifically in cytokine-codifying genes, which will be discussed in the sequence.

Heritable Influences on Cytokine Responses and Bone Loss

Studies suggest that as much as 50% of the risk of disease could be determined by genetic factors [79], and that at least 10–20 disease modifying genes may be involved in the pathogenesis of periodontal diseases [80]. Functional common single nucleotide polymorphisms (SNPs) in genes involved in the initiation, effectuation and control of the host inflammatory immune response have been considered candidate genes in periodontal diseases genetics studies [79-82]. Indeed, heritable differences in cytokines production can result in phenotypes prone to develop different types and degrees of immune-inflammatory reactions, and accordingly, genetic variations have been associated with the resistance or susceptibility to periodontal diseases [83]. In accordance, knockout mice models demonstrate a cause-and-effect relationship between different pro- and anti-inflammatory cytokines and the signs of experimental periodontitis [43, 45, 84]. However, one may argue that knockout mice models represent an extreme situation were a given cytokine is completely absent, and therefore not properly mimetize the putative effect of genetic variations that could account for the individual variations seen in human disease. Alternatively, it was previously demonstrated that two mice strains genetically selected for maximum (AIRmax) or minimum (AIRmin) inflammatory reaction [85-89], present a very distinct phenotype upon experimental PD induction. AIRmax mice infected with A. actinomycetemcomitans exhibit a significantly increased inflammatory cell migration and the alveolar bone resorption when compared to the AIRmin strain [90]. However, although animal models confirm a high degree of heritability and clear genotype/phenotype correlations [90-91], the results of human studies of periodontal disease are inconsistent and controversial [79-80, 92].

Heritable differences are reported in IL-1β production, and SNPs, specially the T allele in the IL1B+3954 loci, have been associated with increased cytokine production [3, 6, 41]. Indeed, studies have indicated a role for such polymorphism in the risk assessment for diverse inflammatory diseases due the increased IL-1β production [3, 7, 41, 52]. Regarding periodontal disease, while some studies demonstrate that subjects with the IL1B+3954 T allele have an increased risk for developing severe periodontitis, other studies were not able to demonstrate such association [12, 17, 27, 48]. In a previous investigation [47], our group demonstrated that similar frequencies of IL1B+3954 SNP were found in PD and control groups, and was found to be associated with increased transcriptional levels of IL-1β [47]. Accordingly, IL1B SNP +3954 was the first polymorphism associated with PDs susceptibility [16, 22], resulting in the development of commercial genetic tests for risk assessment to PDs.

Similarly, heritable differences are reported in TNF-α production, particularly the G to A transition at -308 position, was demonstrated to affect the binding of transcription factors increasing TNF-α production up to five fold *in vitro,* and also to be associated with increased cytokine levels *in vivo* [93-94]. Therefore, the TNFA-308 A allele have been associated with increased risk for the development of diverse infectious and inflammatory diseases [95-97]. Indeed, TNFA-308 A allele was demonstrated to be associated with higher levels of TNF-α production by oral PMN from patients with adult periodontitis [98] and with the severity of chronic periodontitis [99]. Regarding TNFA-308G/A SNP, we previously demonstrated that no statistically significant differences were found in the frequency of TNFA-308 SNP in control and PD groups, in spite of the higher frequency of A allele in CP group; and also a positive association between TNFA-308 A allele and TNF-α mRNA transcriptional levels was demonstrated [48].

The potential genetic influence can also affect IL-10 production. Indeed, studies demonstrated a high individual variation in the levels of IL-10 in diseased periodontal tissues, and such range is thought to be significant in the determination of disease outcome [2,10,11]. Moreover, heritable differences are reported in IL-10 production, and several polymorphic sequences have been identified in the IL-10 gene promoter [12-14]. Three SNPs in the IL-10 gene promoter (−1082 G/A, −819 C/T, −592 C/A) show strong linkage disequilibrium and form two common haplotypes, designated as ATA and GCChaplotypes. Therefore, due to the linkage disequilibrium the presence of these haplotypes can be fully determined by the analysis of the −592 C/A polymorphism, where the occurrence of the A allele indicates the presence of the ATAhaplotype [15,16]. The ATA haplotype has been associated with decreased synthesis of IL-10 in vitro and in vivo [13,17,18], and is frequently associated with pathological conditions [19,20]. In this scenario, we previously demonstrated that IL-10 promoter -592C/A SNP, was associated with lower levels of IL-10, TIMP-3 and OPG mRNA expression in diseased periodontal tissues, and were also associated with disease severity as mean pocket dept [46]. Interestingly, such study demonstrate that IL10-592 SNP is functional in CP, being associated with lower levels of IL-10 mRNA expression, which is supposed to consequently decrease the expression of the downstream genes TIMP-3 and OPG, and influence bone loss levels and PD outcome [46].

At this point, a very intriguing question arise: if functional SNPs modulate the expression of cytokines clearly involved in PD pathogenesis, why the results of genetic studies of human studies of periodontal disease are so highly inconsistent and controversial [79-80, 92]? Among the possible explanations for the divergences between various studies, it would be reasonable to list: genetic variations among different ethnic groups evaluated, studies with a limited number of individuals, variations in the criteria for selection of the experimental groups, and especially the absence of evaluation of covariates that influence the development of PDs [83, 100-101].

In this scenario, it is important to consider one of the PD peculiarities: the type of microbial exposure that triggers disease development. In general infectious diseases genetics studies where a target genetic variant is investigated in a cases and controls sampled from a given endemic area [102]. However, in periodontitis context, the control of microbial biofilm by simple oral hygiene procedures eliminates the natural exposure to the disease etiologic factor, and consequently the determination of the susceptibility/resistance phenotypes is impaired. Indeed, an essential point to be considered is the existence of susceptible and resistant groups to development of PDs. Despite all possible variations associated to clinical phenotypes definition [time of establishment, severity and patterns of disease progression], the existence of susceptible individuals to the development of PDs is unquestionable. Indeed, different forms of periodontal disease affect a majority of the population, and more than 70% of individuals can be considered susceptible to development of periodontitis, in different degrees [1-2, 6, 103]. However, the definition of individuals' potentially genetically resistant group to development of PDs is extremely complex. As previously mentioned, the selection of periodontal healthy subjects to compose the control group, invariably used in genetic association studies related to the PDs, does not necessarily reflect the genetic resistance to disease development, but usually reflects the adequate control of risk factors by individuals in this group. Thus, in a simplistic view, we can consider that the experimental group is composed of 100% of susceptible individuals, while only 30% of control subjects are potentially resistant. Considering also the relatively low frequency of SNPs routinely investigated, the possibility of detecting a statistically significant association is really slight. Then, classic genetic association approaches applied to periodontal disease have a greater tendency to result in false negative results, ruling out the putative role of specific SNPs in the PDs pathogenesis. In fact, the majority of attempts to correlate SNPs with susceptibility/resistance to PDs resulted in negative results [22, 83, 100-101, 104-106].

A recent study of our group [107] demonstrates that the periodontally healthy population presents intermediate genotypic characteristics between chronic periodontitis and chronic gingivitis groups, which reflect its heterogeneous mixed nature. Also, such investigation demonstrated that the observation of the exposure concept from the microbial viewpoint significantly impacts the odds of identification of genetic factors involved [or not] in periodontitis pathogenesis when compared with the traditional case-control approach [107]. Accordingly, the phenotype definition is crucial in designing any genetic study, especially an association study, and previous studies report that the power of a study depends heavily on the phenotype measured and that misclassification or measurement error can dramatically reduce the power [108-111]. Also, the adequate group selection focused on extreme phenotypes minimizes phenotypic heterogeneity and can improve statistical power particularly when sample size is limited due to technical or financial constraints [108-109, 112-115].

Despite the controversies of genetic association previously described, considering the biological feasibility of the SNPs associations previously found, and using data from our group as an example [107], alleles/genotypes associated with a hyperresponsive phenotype (i.e. IL1B-3954-T, TNFA-308-A) were more prevalent in the PD group, while hyporesponsive SNPs [IL10-592-C] prevailed in the 'periodontitis-resistant' cohort [107]. As previously mentioned, these SNPs have been demonstrated as functional in both in vivo and in vitro studies [79, 82-83, 116], and could account for the differences in the nature of host response and distinct outcomes of chronic gingivitis and chronic periodontitis [39, 117]. Therefore, the presence of a hyperresponsive SNP can be interpreted as a risk factor for chronic periodontitis, while its absence or consequently the presence of the respective hyporesponsive SNP in chronic gingivitis cohort may represent a protective factor [107]. However, a valid criticism is this approach is that periodontitis- 'resistant' and 'susceptible' subjects are exposed to distinct microbial profiles and that major periodontopathogens may directly interfere with the local immunoregulatory network. As previously mentioned, bacteria are essential (but not sufficient) in the pathogenesis of periodontitis, quantitative and qualitative microbial features do not necessarily correlate with disease incidence and severity [21, 79, 118]. However, specific periodontopathogens can specifically modulate some cytokines also modulated by the above mentioned SNPs, and therefore the potential microbial impact in cytokine modulation and the consequent bone loss will be discussed in the sequence.

Microbial Influences on Cytokine Responses and Bone Loss

Regardless of the genetic profile, the presence of microorganisms remain be considered as an essential factor for the development of PDs. It should be remembered that, even in the absence of classics periodontopathogens, the accumulation of gram-negative bacteria in subgingival biofilm could also lead to the development of PDs. The LPS, the main structural component of the cell wall of Gram-negative bacteria, is considered as the immunodominant antigen expressed by periodontal pathogens and typically results in a potent immune and inflammatory response by activation of Toll like receptors (TLRs).

Obviously, the role of microorganisms goes beyond the TLR- signaling pathway. Several factors seem to be involved in this context such as: virulence factors of pathogens, stimulation by toxins or superantigens, ability to escape the immune response that contributes to chronicity of the response or facilitate the colonization of the biofilm by other microorganisms, increasing the bacterial load and the diversity of antigenic stimuli in the environment periodontal. These factors are associated with increased severity of periodontal disease.

Accordingly, the red complex periodontopathogens (i.e. *Porphyromonas gingivalis*, *Tannerella forsythia* and *Treponema denticola*) and A. actinomycetemcomitans characteristically induce IL-1β expression [2, 23]. It is also important to consider that the presence of specific periodontopathogens could also contribute to the modulation of IL-1β levels. In fact, *P. gingivalis, T. forsythia and T. denticola* positive sites were found to present a significant higher expression of IL-1β when compared to the negative ones. In accordance, *P. gingivalis* can induce IL-1β production by diverse cell types, and was also associated with increased IL-1β levels in periodontal lesions [119-122]. Similarly, *T. forsythia and T. denticola* have been associated with IL-1β production *in vitro* and *in vivo* [121-123]. Complementarily, *P. gingivalis, T. forsythia and T. denticola* were associated with higher scores of disease severity parameters, in accordance with previous studies [12, 121-122, 124]. Interestingly, the analysis of red complex periodontopathogens individually and as group resulted in similar results, probably due their simultaneous occurrence in most of the patients. Indeed, the red complex periodontopathogens were shown to exist as consortium [125-127], and to exhibit synergistic virulence in a rat model of polymicrobial periodontal infection [128]. In accordance, previous investigations of our group demonstrate an increase of IL-1β levels associated with the simultaneous occurrence of 2 or 3 red complex species, suggesting an increase of pathogenic pro-inflammatory role for these bacteria [47]. On the other hand, *A. actinomycetemcomitans* were not correlated with IL-1β expression [47]. While some studies describes that *A. actinomycetemcomitans* increase IL-1β production in vitro [129-130], others describe that their virulence factors can inhibits inflammatory cytokine production [131-132]. It is important to consider that in spite of *A. actinomycetemcomitans* be sometimes detected in CP sites, it is more prevalent in aggressive periodontitis [133].

Similarly to described to IL-1, the red complex periodontopathogens *and A. actinomycetemcomitans* characteristically induce TNF-α production [134-135]. It is also important to consider that the presence of specific periodontopathogens also could modulate TNF-α levels. In fact, *P. gingivalis, T. forsythia and T. denticola* positive sites presented a significant higher expression of TNF-α when compared to the negative ones, and its loads were positively correlated with TNF-α mRNA levels. In accordance, *P. gingivalis* can induce TNF-α production by diverse cell types [134-136], and was also associated with TNF-α levels in periodontal lesions [121, 137]. Indeed, TNF-α mediates *P. gingivalis*-induced bone resorption in mice [138]. Similarly, *T. forsythia and T. denticola* have been associated with TNF-α production *in vitro* and *in vivo* [121, 123]. Complementarily, *P. gingivalis, T. forsythia and T. denticola* were associated with higher scores of disease severity parameters, in accordance with previous studies [12, 47, 124]. Interestingly, the evaluations of red complex periodontopathogens detection individually resulted in similar results, probably due their simultaneous occurrence in the majority of the patients. Indeed, the red complex periodontopathogens were shown to exist as consortium [127], and to exhibit synergistic virulence in a rat model of polymicrobial periodontal infection [128]. In a previous investigation, our group demonstrated a gradual increase in TNF-α levels associated with the simultaneous occurrence of red complex species, suggesting a synergistic pathogenic pro-inflammatory role for these bacteria [48]. On the other hand, *A. actinomycetemcomitans* positive sites presented a slight decrease in TNF-α expression, but such difference did not reach the statistical significance [48]. While some studies describe that *A. actinomycetemcomitans* can induce TNF-α production *in vitro* and *in vivo* [135, 139], others describe that *A. actinomycetemcomitans* presents immunosuppressive properties that could inhibit this inflammatory cytokine production [140-142].

While the aggressive periodontitis associated pathogen *A. actinomycetemcomitans* association with the expression of pro-inflammatory cytokines remain controversial, extremely interesting results may suggest more complexes associations between pathogens and host response rather than basic response amplification. While similar levels of IL-1β were found in positive and negative sites for *A. actinomycetemcomitans*, a trend [not statistically significant] the lower expression of TNF-α was observed in sites positive for A. actinomycetemcomitans [48]. Indeed, some studies revealed that *A. actinomycetemcomitans* can induce the production of proinflammatory cytokines *in vitro* and *in vivo* [135, 139], however other authors described that virulence factors of this pathogen may inhibit such response [132, 140, 142-143]. These new findings, although potentially controversial [host response attenuation by a periodontopathogen associated with severe periodontal tissue destruction], can be considered as a progress in the study of virulence factors of classics periodontopathogens. In fact, a new generation of studies has made significant advances concerning to the microbial aspect of the PDs. In this context, the detection of several viruses in periodontal biofilm may be the most interesting discovery [144-145]. Viruses such as HSV (*herpes simplex virus*), HCMV [*human cytomegalovirus*] and EBV (*Epstein-Barr virus*) have been related to increased periodontopathogens classics frequency and load, especially the red complex periodontopathogens [146]. The high frequency of virus in periodontal lesions has suggested a reinterpretation of the immunopathogenesis of PDs; however the mechanisms by which viruses could affect the PDs pathogenesis remain unclear. Some studies suggest that viruses such as HCMV could directly affect the transcription of cytokines (eg IL-1β), increasing periodontal disease severity [147]. Beyond the possible local effects, systemic viral infections, primarily HIV, can lead to pronounced alterations in the host response, and can also be associated with augmentation of disease severity [148].

Recently, HTLV-I (human T-cell lymphotropic virus type-I), a highly pathogenic retrovirus, was also associated with several oral manifestations, including PDs [149-150]. In a previous study, our group demonstrated that the HTLV-I patients presented a higher prevalence and severity of PDs [151]. Indeed, parameters such as bleeding on probing, attachment loss and probing depth were more pronounced in patients seropositive for HTLV-I [151]. Whereas HTLV-I infection leads to the development of motor impairments [152], the first hypothesis about the exacerbation of periodontal disease was related to poor plaque control, impaired by motor difficulties. However, the plaque index in these patients is similar to HTLV-I negative patients, as well as the classics periodontopathogens frequency and load [151]. Evaluations of the cytokines expression pattern in periodontal lesions demonstrated a significant increase in IL-1β, TNF-α [regardless of the genotypes of IL1B +3954 and TNFA-308] and IFN-γ, while lower levels of IL- 10 were detected in the HTLV-I positive patients. It was also verified that FOXP3 levels, a surface marker of regulatory T cells, were strongly reduced in these patients [151]. In fact, it is possible that such consequences of HTLV-I are due by an uncontrolled systemic expression of cytokines, triggered by the lack of regulatory T cell function, as a result of viral infection [152-155]. Therefore, the presence of a usual microbial stimulus, similar to HTLV-I seronegative patients, impairs in the control of immunoregulation by the lack of regulatory T cells results in a significantly exacerbated response and increased tissue destruction.

At this point, it is possible to describe the association of individual pathogens, or some microbial clusters such as the red complex, with interesting variations in the pattern of cytokines produced locally, which in turn affect the bone loss outcome at periodontal lesions. However, it is noteworthy that very similar associations were previously accounted for the influence of functional SNPs, so a clear potential overlapping modulation scenario is suggested. Based on the experience of using an experimental model in which intend to minimize or isolate variables, it is important to apply this idea to human PDs, creating strategies to control the possible influence of some variables and enable the development of studies with highly specific and limited aims. Therefore, in the sequence some studies aimed to isolate some variables and unravel the individual and combined role of microbes and SNPs in the modulation of PDs severity will be considered.

Are Genetic and Microbial Influences on Cytokine Responses Overlaping or Independent Modulators?

Among the variables involved in the pathogenesis of periodontal disease, it is possible to list: microbial factors, the host genetic background and the nature of its inflammatory immune response raised against the microbes, and local modifying factors (including local factors such as overhanging restorations, malpositioned teeth), environmental factors (especially smoking) and systemic factors (such as comorbidities, which will be discussed afterward) [15, 21-26, 100]. In order to unravel the individual role of potential factor involved in PD pathogenesis, it is reasonable to suggest that this only can be possible considering initially all the factors independently.

Following this rationale, some studies were drawn in order to identify the influence of specific functional SNPs and classics periodontopathogens such as bacteria of the red complex e *A. actinomycetemcomitans* in the determination of cytokine levels in periodontal tissues and PD outcome. The IL1B+3954 SNP CT and TT genotypes, as well P. gingivalis, T. forsythia and T. denticola, were found to be associated with higher IL-1β levels and with higher values of the clinical parameters of disease severity [47]. Interestingly, concomitant analyses demonstrate that IL1B+3954 and the red complex periodontopathogens were found to independently and additively modulate the levels of IL-1β in periodontal tissues. Similarly, the concurrent presence of both factors was associated with increased scores of disease severity. IL1B+3954 genotypes and red complex periodontopathogens, individually and additively, modulate the levels of IL-1β in diseased tissues of non-smokers chronic periodontitis patients, and consequently, are potentially involved in the determination of disease outcome. In this perspective, IL1B +3954 SNP and red complex bacteria were associated with levels of IL-1β mRNA, independently and additively. Initially, such scenario might be considered predictable or obvious, but since these factors can modulate the expression of IL-1β, independent or additive modulation was unknown. Thus, considering only those variables (the IL1B +3954 SNP and red complex bacteria), it is possible to suppose that both genetic susceptibility in presence of polymorphic T allele as environmental influences (red complex bacteria) can potentially lead to similar levels of IL-1β, contributing to the development of periodontitis at similar levels. Finally, when both variables are present, a more intense inflammatory response is observed in patients genetically predisposed to periodontal disease development (in presence of T allele of the IL1B +3954 SNP). Especially when exposed to virulent pathogens, an additive effect on IL-1β is detected, and virtually can be noticed in increased severity of periodontitis. It should be noted that red complex periodontopathogens frequency and load are similar in different IL1B SNP +3954 genotypes, eliminating a possible confounding factor in this analysis. Considering the occurrence of T allele (CT + TT genotypes), it was observed the frequency of approximately 40%, while the frequency of patients positive for *P. gingivalis* was approximately 75%. Thus, it is possible to consider that, in terms of population, the presence of bacteria could potentially be responsible for an increased number of cases of periodontitis when compared to the T allele of the IL1B +3954 SNP. In addition to this association based on the frequency, evaluating in a general context (analyzing the genotype without considering the presence of periodontopathogens, and vice versa), an increase of approximately 40% was verified in IL-1β in individuals positive for T allele, while individuals positive for *P. gingivalis* showed a 65% increase in the expression levels of IL-1β mRNA. Then, these results suggest that, in addition to potentially being responsible for several cases of periodontitis, the presence of *P. gingivalis* seems to be responsible for more severe cases of the disease, considering that the levels of IL-1β levels are directly associated to tissue damage. However, concerning to the possible clinical impact of such variation, the magnitude of this difference in the probing depth and attachment loss are less pronounced when compared with mRNA levels, respectively 10% and 12% for IL1B +3954 SNPs, and 19% and 34% for *P. gingivalis*. However, the occurrence of an association between genotype and environment resulting in an additive effect is not a general rule. The concomitant analyses of genotypes and periodontopathogens demonstrate that TNFA-308 GA/AA genotypes and the red complex periodontopathogens are independently associated with increased TNF-α levels in periodontal tissues [48]. However, no additive effect was seen when both factors were present. P. gingivalis, T. forsythia, T. denticola counts were positively correlated with TNF-α mRNA expression [48]. Considering that TNFA-308 SNP is functional in several cases, a result similar to IL1B +3954 SNP could be expected, but a possible additive effect was absent suggesting that both factors can lead to a plateau of maximum TNF-α expression[48]. Thus, the regulation of TNF-α expression, both genetic susceptibility (conferred by allele A of TNFA SNP-308) as the environmental influences (presence of red complex) may contribute independently and the same intensity for maximum production of TNF-α.

Therefore, genetic (IL1B+3954, TNF-308 and IL10-592) and microbial (the red complex periodontopathogens) factors can significantly contribute to the immunoregulation of periodontal lesions, influencing periodontitis establishment and progression. However, if one person has IL1B +3954 T allele (deleterious) and IL10-592 C (protector), the effect of both would be canceled, resulting in a neutral vector concerning to the intensity of the response? Indeed, current knowledge about the haplotype-phenotype association is extremely limited, even in highly complex situations such as PDs, which involves multiple microorganisms and several other cofactors [156-157]. Whereas the evaluation of gene-gene interaction are extremely complex, requiring a very large sample size so in order to provide reliable conclusions [157] - the addition of all the variables related to PDs analysis seem to be impractical at this time.

Modifying Factors: Focus on Comorbidities

Besides genetic and microbial factors, co-morbidities appear as important modulators of host response and bone loss outcome associated to PDs. Recent studies demonstrate a parallel development of distinct disorders called co-morbidity, and suggest that similar immunopathogenetic pathways operate in pathogenesis of such parallel disorders [158-160]. The development of regulated immune responses is essential in the host defense against harmful antigens and in the balance between tolerance and immunity to other antigens. Immune-related disorders are the result of inappropriate destruction of normal tissue by unbalanced immune inflammatory reactions, and comprise autoimmune (a failure of the immune self-tolerance mechanism) and inflammatory disorders (an excessive inflammatory reaction in to exogenous antigens) [159]. The possible common pathways responsible for inappropriate or excessive immune response include: genetic factors, such as the human leukocyte antigen (HLA) genes and SNPs; innate and adaptive immune regulation processes and environmental factors, such as infections or dietary components [158-160]. Among the conditions listed as comorbidities that can greatly influence PD outcome, we can list diabetes, rheumatoid arthritis and more recently, allergy/asthma; which will be considered individually in the sequence.

Rheumatoid Arthritis and PD Comorbidity: Genetic and Functional Associations

Results from clinical studies point toward a co-morbidity association between chronic periodontitis and rheumatoid arthritis (RA)[161,162-164]. Such clinical investigations demonstrate that RA can increase the incidence and severity of PD independently or only partially dependent on oral hygiene status or modifying factors [161, 162-167]. RA is a chronic autoimmune inflammatory disease, which possibly arises due to a failure in thymic selection or in the peripheral tolerance mechanisms. RA is characterized by persistent synovial inflammation and progressive destruction of cartilage and bone in the joints [168]. Interestingly, PD and RA share common immunopathogenic mechanisms as the chronic inflammatory reaction associated with soft and mineralized tissue destruction. Indeed, pro-inflammatory (TNF-α, IL-1β), Th1- (IFN-γ) and Th17- (IL-17A) type cytokines are widely expressed in both diseased synovial and periodontal tissue [14, 168]. Furthermore, in both diseases these cytokines present a catabolic role over the tissues, mediated by the production of MMPs and the osteoclastogenic factor RANKL [14, 18, 31, 43, 165-166, 168-170]. Recent studies suggest that the PD and RA interaction can be bi-directional, since the control of periodontal infection reduces the severity of RA [171-172] and the treatment of RA results in clinical benefits to periodontal conditions [36, 173].

In this scenario, a major unanswered question is how a joint lesion could influence the host response at periodontal environment affecting periodontitis outcome. Among the hypothesis raised, considering the common immune and inflammatory features of both diseases, conceptual models link both diseases by causal and noncausal pathways [165-166, 169, 174-176]. Noncausal hypothesis considers that environmental or host factors increase susceptibility to both RA and PD, while causal assumption is that RA and PD can actively interfere with the pathogenesis of each other [165-166, 169, 176]. Noncausal theory is supported by studies demonstrating that the genetic factors implicated in PD can also act as susceptibility factors for RA [165-166]. Genome-wide association studies confirm the clinical observations regarding the co-morbidity of immune-related diseases, and describe the existence of shared genetic susceptibility clusters, involving general immune pathways of T-cell differentiation, T-cell signaling and the innate immune response [159]. Some experimental studies reinforce the noncausal shared genetic susceptibility hypothesis since mice strains share the susceptibility or resistance phenotype to both chronic models arthritis and periodontitis [47, 85, 87-89]. On the other hand, the causal theory is supported by the increased levels of proinflammatory and tissue destructive mediators in the periodontal tissues of RA patients or rodents submitted to experimental RA induction [164, 177-178].

Interestingly, specific pathogens such as *A. actinomycetemcomitans* [179-180] and *P. gingivalis* [181-182] are supposed to play a possible causal role in RA pathogenesis. Indeed, oral bacterial DNAs were found in synovial fluid of RA patients, suggesting that oral pathogens could have a perpetuating effect in joint disease [183]. In addition, numerous infectious agents, including periodontal bacteria, and antibodies against them, have been implicated as contributory to the etiology of RA [166, 184-185]. In this regard, the hypothesis that *P. gingivalis* allows PD patients to be exposed to citrullinated antigens and, consequently, leads to the development of anti-citrullinated peptide antibodies, a predisposing to the risk for RA [169]. *P. gingivalis* expresses the enzyme peptidylarginine deaminase which may modify the amino acid arginine of host protein into the amino acid citrulline. This modification might induce the loss of self-tolerance through the production of antipeptidyl citrulline antibodies by the host, which are known, along with rheumatoid factors, to predate the onset of RA [186-188].

Conversely, a functional interference in the host response against periodontopathogens by RA was verified by our group in a previous study [176]. It was demonstrated that the inflammatory immune response along experimental PD was not only amplified (even higher levels of pro-inflammatory cytokines IL-1β and TNF-α) by RA parallel induction, but also was skewed toward a Th1 and Th17 response (increased IFN-γ and IL-17 levels). Considering that the lymph nodes environment play a central role in orchestrating the adaptive immune response, which include the polarization of naïve T cells into characteristic Th subsets, it was demonstrated that the induction of RA resulted in significant changes of the submandibular lymph nodes (the major draining LNs of oral cavity) environment, being the levels of Tbet and RORgamma (the prototypical transcription factors involved in Th1 and Th17 cells polarization) significantly increased [176]. Therefore, it is possible to consider that a systemic immune activation due RA skews the polarization of Th cells into Th1- and Th17-type. Other possible mechanism involved in the upregulation of innate responsiveness, since the induction of RA also resulted in increased levels of inflammatory cytokine TNF-α in the serum [176]. Indeed, data from our group demonstrated that anti-TNF-α therapy prevented arthritis and PD development [175]. Furthermore, the anti-TNF-α therapy reversed the Th polarization patterns associated with arthritis-induced PD (predominantly Th17) [175] and with exacerbation of infection-induced PD by arthritis (predominantly Th1) (unpublished data).

Besides its role in the exacerbation of PD, RA was described to co-induce PDs [169, 176]. In the co-induction scenario, the unbalanced immune response due RA development triggers periodontitis development in response to the commensal subgingival microbiota, which in standard homeostatic conditions would not be harmful to the host [169]. In fact, such hypothesis was recently confirmed in two distinct experimental models [175-176]. In the pristane-induced RA model (PIA) [176] mice that received pristane injection but were not submitted to the deliberate induction of periodontitis (i.e. oral inoculation of periodontopathogens or placement of ligatures) developed a significant alveolar bone loss. Interestingly, the control of normal oral microbiota abrogated PIA-induced alveolar bone loss. Therefore, it is possible to suggest that for the leukocyte migration triggered by the normal oral biofilm, when associated with altered immune responsiveness due to experimental RA, results in alveolar bone loss even in the absence of classic periodontopathogens. These finding support the hypothesis that RA could co-induce and just not exacerbate PD [169]. This hypothesis was also reinforced in an antigen-induced arthritis [AIA] model [175] where AIA was spontaneously associated with inflammatory signs of PD, without any manipulation of the oral environment. In this model, the Ag challenge of the knee joint rapidly triggered signs of PD, characterized by alveolar bone loss; osteoclast differentiation; and an increase in the levels of MPO, proinflammatory cytokines, and RANKL. The most interesting point is that

AIA differs from PIA and other experimental RA models because the trigger point is local rather than systemic, i.e. generalized systemic inflammation is not present after immunization. Despite the local joint challenge, AIA triggered a low-grade systemic inflammation measured by increased serum levels of C-reactive protein, production of anti-collagen antibodies, and hyper responsiveness to periodontal proteins, such as the collagen I. This systemic imbalance might respond for the connection between the joint and the periodontal conditions observed. In agreement with previous data, co-induction of PD by AIA only happened in cooperation with the oral microbiota, which clearly demonstrates the need of 'two hits' to induce a secondary disease [169].

Therefore, the mentioned studies support the two-hit model, where the presence of a "suitable" environment, such as the mouth with its commensal microbiota (first hit), along with the systemic immunoactivated milieu triggered by RA (i.e., autoantibodies, Th polarization, and release of acute-phase proteins; second hit) results in inflammatory cell influx and alveolar bone loss, even in the absence of classic periodontopathogens or greater amounts of dental plaque [175-176]. In this setting, it is suggested that the interaction between PD and RA involves a shared susceptibility genotype prone to hyper inflammatory responsiveness and functional interferences comprising the amplification of innate immunity and a skewed adaptive response. Interestingly, a similar pattern of interference on and even co-induction of PDs is described to the co-morbidity with diabetes, which will be discussed in the sequence. Similarly, experimental diabetes in rats triggers, or co-induces, the onset of alterations that are typical of periodontal diseases even in the absence of aggressive factors such as ligatures or inoculation of classic periodontopathogens [189].

Diabetes and PD Comorbidity: A RAGE Mediated Process

Diabetes mellitus represents a spectrum of metabolic disorders characterized by abnormally high levels of glucose in the blood. Indeed, hyperglycemia is the hallmark of diabetes mellitus, being associated with several acute and chronic complications such as nephropathy, neuropathy, retinopathy and cardiovascular diseases [190]. Among the pathologies triggered or exacerbated by diabetes, the effect of chronic hyperglycemic in periodontal environment has been characterized by an increase in periodontitis prevalence and severity. In this way, periodontal disease has been termed the sixth complication of diabetes [191-192].

The establishment and severity of these diabetic complications are strikingly related to the formation of advanced glycation end products (AGEs) that occur in presence of hyperglycemia [193-194]. The interaction between AGEs with their specific receptors RAGE triggers an exacerbated inflammatory response, characterized by increased expression of inflammatory mediators, osteoclastogenic factors and MMPs [193-194]. In fact, treatment with soluble RAGE, the extracellular ligand-binding domain of RAGE that antagonizes the interaction of ligands with the whole receptor, resulted in decreased cytokines and matrix MMPs levels in gingival tissues, accompanied by inhibition of alveolar bone loss in a dose-dependent manner in diabetic animals [195]. Therefore, AGE–RAGE interaction leads to the exacerbated inflammatory response to the bacterial challenge, resulting in subsequent increased tissue destruction. In addition, it has been also suggested suggest that diabetes interfere in host defense mechanisms such as chemotaxis, adherence, phagocytosis and apoptosis, contributing to tissue destruction [196-197].

Thus, the presence of diabetes renders a previously resistant host into a susceptible phenotype, thus triggering the development of periodontal disease. Consequently, diabetes can be considered a very important risk factor to periodontal disease since it could also trigger, or even co-induce the onset of periodontal disease, and not only exacerbate the established disease [169, 189]. In the general context, diabetes seems to be associated with host response dysfunction, which exacerbates the expression and/or activation of intracellular signaling molecules, resulting in upregulation of inflammatory mediators. Therefore, diabetes may trigger periodontal disease induction throughout the deregulation of immune and inflammatory response against commensal periodopathogenic microbiota.

Allergic Disease and PD Comorbidity: The Opposing Scenario

While clinical studies describe the co-morbidity of PD with diabetes and RA as factors that increase the severity of PD and the bone loss, diseases associated with opposing immunological patterns may present an inverse association [161, 192] [162-164, 176]. While similar patterns of immune response may converge to amplify the severity of certain co-morbid conditions, diseases associated with opposing immunological patterns may present an inverse association. Two wide epidemiological studies demonstrate an inverse association between periodontitis and oral pathogens with allergic disease (AL) [198, 199]. In immunological terms, it sounds reasonable to conceive that diseases characterized by the production of distinct and mutually inhibitory cytokines present an inverse association. This paradigm fits in the "hygiene hypothesis", which postulates that the immune response raised against infections may have protective effects against the allergies development [200-201]. While cross-sectional data from human studies [198] [199] does not allow a direct cause-effect association, a recent experimental study demonstrate that subcutaneous infection with a periodontal pathogen attenuate airway allergic inflammation [202]. In a previous study, our group experimentally confirmed the inverse clinical association between PD and AL described in clinical studies [203]. The AL/PD interaction involves functional immunological interferences comprising alterations in the patterns of T cell transcription factors expression in LN environment and modulation of local host response in periodontium. Interestingly, opposing the finding previously mentioned related to PD/diabetes and PD/RA co-morbidity scenarios, the co induction of allergy is characterized by decreased bone loss due a lower production of TNF-α, IL-1β, IFN-γ and IL-17A, and a trend toward higher IL-4 production in allergic mice submitted to the induction of experimental PD[203]. IL-4, the Th2-prototypical cytokine, suppresses the polarization of Th1 cells and Th17 cells and its signature cytokines production [204-208]. In fact, IL-4 production in periodontal tissues of allergic mice parallel with the downregulation of IFN-γ and IL-17, previously mentioned as mediators of osteolytic process in periodontal lesions. Indeed, IL-4 is also able to interfere in the MMPs/TIMPs and RANKL/OPG ratios [209-210] [211], reinforcing its potential protective role. Regarding the mechanistic basis of the attenuation of bone loss along experimental PD in allergic mice, it was demonstrated that the transcription factor GATA3 [Th2-related] expression levels were significantly increased while Tbet (Th1-related) and RORγ (Th17-related) were decreased in allergic mice [203]. Interestingly, such modulation comprises an inverse pattern of the situation triggered by the co-induction of RA [176].

Considering in summary all the comorbidities scenarios described here, the occurrence of co-morbidity is associated with convergent similar immunopathogenetic pathways, while conditions presenting opposing patterns of immune response may present an antagonistic effect [158-160, 212]. Indeed, diabetes, rheumatoid arthritis and inflammatory intestinal disease are described as conditions where the production of pro-inflammatory, Th1- and Th17-type cytokines is prominent, while airway allergy is usually characterized by a Th2 biased response [161, 162-164]. However, direct comparisons with PD must be careful in the view of the complex and still unclear role of T helper subsets in PD pathogenesis previously discussed [17, 213]. Also, the modulation of innate immunity related mechanisms is also an important feature of the comorbidity scenario, and such modulation can be dependent or independent of subsequent adaptive response.

SUMMARY/CONCLUDING REMARKS

Taken together, it is well established that periodontitis is caused by an unbalanced host response to periodontopathogens. However, despite the presence of bacteria is required, it is not sufficient to trigger periodontitis, demonstrating that the host response is an essential step to establishment and progression of periodontal disease. Based in these findings, it is reasonable to consider the involvement of inflammatory and immune mechanisms in the pathogenesis of this disease. In fact, periodontal disease is mainly characterized by bone resorption, resulting in alveolar bone loss, demonstrating a close relationship between immune system and bone metabolism. Beyond these factors, the influence of genetic factors, especially single nucleotides polymorphisms (SNPs) also affect the severity of periodontitis. However, the real role of each factor as well their interaction are complex and requires further research to unravel the putative mechanisms involved in this increased prevalence and severity of periodontal disease in presence of such factors.

These studies will certainly contribute to the development of new strategies concerning to periodontitis treatment, considering that the current treatment of this pathology is mainly based in mechanical procedures. Considering that periodontitis is a multifactorial disease, it would be reasonable that preventive and therapeutic strategies also engage immune and genetic factors. Although the difficulty to specify the targets, this idea needs to be evaluated with more attention in order to improve the diagnostic and treatment of periodontal disease.

References

[1] Brown LJ, Loe H. Prevalence, extent, severity and progression of periodontal disease. *Periodontology 2000*. 1993 Jun;2:57-71.

[2] Loe H, Anerud A, Boysen H, Morrison E. Natural history of periodontal disease in man. Rapid, moderate and no loss of attachment in Sri Lankan laborers 14 to 46 years of age. *Journal of clinical periodontology*. 1986 May;13(5):431-45.

[3] The pathogenesis of periodontal diseases. *Journal of periodontology*. 1999 Apr;70(4):457-70.

[4] Kinane DF, Attstrom R. Advances in the pathogenesis of periodontitis. Group B consensus report of the fifth European Workshop in Periodontology. *Journal of clinical periodontology*. 2005;32 Suppl 6:130-1.

[5] Kinane D, Bouchard P. Periodontal diseases and health: Consensus Report of the Sixth European Workshop on Periodontology. *Journal of clinical periodontology*. 2008 Sep;35(8 Suppl):333-7.

[6] Consensus report. Periodontal diseases: epidemiology and diagnosis. *Annals of periodontology / the American Academy of Periodontology*. 1996 Nov;1(1):216-22.

[7] Nanci A, Bosshardt DD. Structure of periodontal tissues in health and disease. *Periodontology 2000*. 2006;40:11-28.

[8] Clark WB, Loe H. Mechanisms of initiation and progression of periodontal disease. *Periodontology 2000*. 1993 Jun;2:72-82.

[9] Feng Z, Weinberg A. Role of bacteria in health and disease of periodontal tissues. *Periodontology 2000*. 2006;40:50-76.

[10] Haffajee AD, Socransky SS. Microbiology of periodontal diseases: introduction. *Periodontology 2000*. 2005;38:9-12.

[11] O'Brien-Simpson NM, Veith PD, Dashper SG, Reynolds EC. Antigens of bacteria associated with periodontitis. *Periodontology 2000*. 2004;35:101-34.

[12] Socransky SS, Haffajee AD. Periodontal microbial ecology. *Periodontology 2000*. 2005;38:135-87.

[13] Cochran DL. Inflammation and bone loss in periodontal disease. *Journal of periodontology*. 2008 Aug;79(8 Suppl):1569-76.

[14] Graves D. Cytokines that promote periodontal tissue destruction. *Journal of periodontology*. 2008 Aug;79(8 Suppl):1585-91.

[15] Van Dyke TE. Inflammation and periodontal diseases: a reappraisal. *Journal of periodontology*. 2008 Aug;79(8 Suppl):1501-2.

[16] Van Dyke TE, Kornman KS. Inflammation and factors that may regulate inflammatory response. *Journal of periodontology*. 2008 Aug;79(8 Suppl):1503-7.
[17] Gaffen SL, Hajishengallis G. A new inflammatory cytokine on the block: re-thinking periodontal disease and the Th1/Th2 paradigm in the context of Th17 cells and IL-17. *Journal of dental research*. 2008 Sep;87(9):817-28.
[18] Graves DT, Cochran D. The contribution of interleukin-1 and tumor necrosis factor to periodontal tissue destruction. *Journal of periodontology*. 2003 Mar;74(3):391-401.
[19] Yamazaki K, Yoshie H, Seymour GJ. T cell regulation of the immune response to infection in periodontal diseases. *Histology and histopathology*. 2003 Jul;18(3):889-96.
[20] Baker PJ. The role of immune responses in bone loss during periodontal disease. *Microbes Infect*. 2000 Aug;2(10):1181-92.
[21] Offenbacher S, Barros SP, Beck JD. Rethinking periodontal inflammation. *Journal of periodontology*. 2008 Aug;79(8 Suppl): 1577-84.
[22] Kornman KS. Mapping the pathogenesis of periodontitis: a new look. *Journal of periodontology*. 2008 Aug;79(8 Suppl):1560-8.
[23] Sanz M, Quirynen M. Advances in the aetiology of periodontitis. Group A consensus report of the 5th European Workshop in Periodontology. *Journal of clinical periodontology*. 2005;32 Suppl 6:54-6.
[24] Williams RC. Understanding and managing periodontal diseases: a notable past, a promising future. *Journal of periodontology*. 2008 Aug;79(8 Suppl):1552-9.
[25] Wilson AG. Epigenetic regulation of gene expression in the inflammatory response and relevance to common diseases. *Journal of periodontology*. 2008 Aug;79(8 Suppl):1514-9.
[26] Nunn ME. Understanding the etiology of periodontitis: an overview of periodontal risk factors. *Periodontology 2000*. 2003;32:11-23.
[27] Baker AH, Edwards DR, Murphy G. Metalloproteinase inhibitors: biological actions and therapeutic opportunities. *Journal of cell science*. 2002 Oct 1;115(Pt 19):3719-27.
[28] Hannas AR, Pereira JC, Granjeiro JM, Tjaderhane L. The role of matrix metalloproteinases in the oral environment. *Acta odontologica Scandinavica*. 2007 Feb;65(1):1-13.
[29] Sorsa T, Tjaderhane L, Salo T. Matrix metalloproteinases (MMPs) in oral diseases. *Oral diseases*. 2004 Nov;10(6):311-8.

[30] Garlet GP, Martins W, Jr., Fonseca BA, Ferreira BR, Silva JS. Matrix metalloproteinases, their physiological inhibitors and osteoclast factors are differentially regulated by the cytokine profile in human periodontal disease. *Journal of clinical periodontology*. 2004 Aug;31(8):671-9.

[31] Garlet GP, Cardoso CR, Silva TA, Ferreira BR, Avila-Campos MJ, Cunha FQ, et al. Cytokine pattern determines the progression of experimental periodontal disease induced by Actinobacillus actinomycetemcomitans through the modulation of MMPs, RANKL, and their physiological inhibitors. *Oral Microbiol. Immunol*. 2006 Feb; 21(1):12-20.

[32] Teitelbaum SL. Bone resorption by osteoclasts. *Science (New York, NY*. 2000 Sep 1;289(5484):1504-8.

[33] Katagiri T, Takahashi N. Regulatory mechanisms of osteoblast and osteoclast differentiation. *Oral diseases*. 2002 May;8(3):147-59.

[34] Takayanagi H, Ogasawara K, Hida S, Chiba T, Murata S, Sato K, et al. T-cell-mediated regulation of osteoclastogenesis by signalling cross-talk between RANKL and IFN-gamma. *Nature*. 2000 Nov 30;408(6812): 600-5.

[35] Takayanagi H. Osteoimmunology: shared mechanisms and crosstalk between the immune and bone systems. *Nat. Rev. Immunol*. 2007 Apr; 7(4):292-304.

[36] Mayer Y, Balbir-Gurman A, Machtei EE. Anti-tumor necrosis factor-alpha therapy and periodontal parameters in patients with rheumatoid arthritis. *Journal of periodontology*. 2009 Sep;80(9):1414-20.

[37] Al-Rasheed A, Scheerens H, Rennick DM, Fletcher HM, Tatakis DN. Accelerated alveolar bone loss in mice lacking interleukin-10. *Journal of dental research*. 2003 Aug;82(8):632-5.

[38] Al-Rasheed A, Scheerens H, Srivastava AK, Rennick DM, Tatakis DN. Accelerated alveolar bone loss in mice lacking interleukin-10: late onset. *Journal of periodontal research*. 2004 Jun;39(3):194-8.

[39] Menezes R, Garlet TP, Letra A, Bramante CM, Campanelli AP, Figueira Rde C, et al. Differential patterns of receptor activator of nuclear factor kappa B ligand/osteoprotegerin expression in human periapical granulomas: possible association with progressive or stable nature of the lesions. *Journal of endodontics*. 2008 Aug; 34(8):932-8.

[40] Zhang X, Teng YT. Interleukin-10 inhibits gram-negative-microbe-specific human receptor activator of NF-kappaB ligand-positive CD4+-Th1-cell-associated alveolar bone loss in vivo. *Infection and immunity*. 2006 Aug;74(8):4927-31.

[41] Sasaki H, Okamatsu Y, Kawai T, Kent R, Taubman M, Stashenko P. The interleukin-10 knockout mouse is highly susceptible to Porphyromonas gingivalis-induced alveolar bone loss. *Journal of periodontal research*. 2004 Dec;39(6):432-41.

[42] Garlet GP. Destructive and protective roles of cytokines in periodontitis: a re-appraisal from host defense and tissue destruction viewpoints. *Journal of dental research*. 2010 Dec;89(12):1349-63.

[43] Garlet GP, Cardoso CR, Campanelli AP, Ferreira BR, Avila-Campos MJ, Cunha FQ, et al. The dual role of p55 tumour necrosis factor-alpha receptor in Actinobacillus actinomycetemcomitans-induced experimental periodontitis: host protection and tissue destruction. *Clin. Exp. Immunol*. 2007 Jan;147(1):128-38.

[44] Roberts L, McColl GJ. Tumour necrosis factor inhibitors: risks and benefits in patients with rheumatoid arthritis. *Internal medicine journal*. 2004 Dec;34(12):687-93.

[45] Alayan J, Ivanovski S, Farah CS. Alveolar bone loss in T helper 1/T helper 2 cytokine-deficient mice. *Journal of periodontal research*. 2007 Apr;42(2):97-103.

[46] Claudino M, Trombone AP, Cardoso CR, Ferreira SB, Jr., Martins W, Jr., Assis GF, et al. The broad effects of the functional IL-10 promoter-592 polymorphism: modulation of IL-10, TIMP-3, and OPG expression and their association with periodontal disease outcome. *J. Leukoc. Biol*. 2008 Dec;84(6):1565-73.

[47] Ferreira SB, Jr., Trombone AP, Repeke CE, Cardoso CR, Martins W, Jr., Santos CF, et al. An interleukin-1beta (IL-1beta) single-nucleotide polymorphism at position 3954 and red complex periodontopathogens independently and additively modulate the levels of IL-1beta in diseased periodontal tissues. *Infection and immunity*. 2008 Aug;76(8):3725-34.

[48] Trombone AP, Cardoso CR, Repeke CE, Ferreira SB, Jr., Martins W, Jr., Campanelli AP, et al. Tumor necrosis factor-alpha -308G/A single nucleotide polymorphism and red-complex periodontopathogens are independently associated with increased levels of tumor necrosis factor-alpha in diseased periodontal tissues. *Journal of periodontal research*. 2009 Oct;44(5):598-608.

[49] Gemmell E, Seymour GJ. Immunoregulatory control of Th1/Th2 cytokine profiles in periodontal disease. *Periodontology 2000*. 2004; 35:21-41.

[50] Teng YT. Mixed periodontal Th1-Th2 cytokine profile in Actinobacillus actinomycetemcomitans-specific osteoprotegerin ligand (or RANK-L)-

mediated alveolar bone destruction in vivo. *Infection and immunity*. 2002 Sep;70(9):5269-73.

[51] Teng YT. The role of acquired immunity and periodontal disease progression. *Crit Rev Oral Biol. Med*. 2003;14(4):237-52.

[52] Berglundh T, Donati M. Aspects of adaptive host response in periodontitis. *Journal of clinical periodontology*. 2005;32 Suppl 6: 87-107.

[53] Garlet GP, Martins W, Jr., Ferreira BR, Milanezi CM, Silva JS. Patterns of chemokines and chemokine receptors expression in different forms of human periodontal disease. *Journal of periodontal research*. 2003 Apr; 38(2):210-7.

[54] Cardoso CR, Garlet GP, Moreira AP, Junior WM, Rossi MA, Silva JS. Characterization of CD4+CD25+ natural regulatory T cells in the inflammatory infiltrate of human chronic periodontitis. *J. Leukoc. Biol.* 2008 Jul;84(1):311-8.

[55] Cardoso CRG, G. P.; Crippa, G.; Rosa, A.; Martins-Jr, W.; Rossi, M.; Silva, J.S. Evidences of the presence of Th17 cells in chronic lesions of human periodontal disease. *Oral Microbiol. Immunol*. 2008;in press.

[56] Belkaid Y, Piccirillo CA, Mendez S, Shevach EM, Sacks DL. CD4+CD25+ regulatory T cells control Leishmania major persistence and immunity. *Nature*. 2002 Dec 5;420(6915):502-7.

[57] Belkaid Y, Rouse BT. Natural regulatory T cells in infectious disease. *Nat. Immunol*. 2005 Apr;6(4):353-60.

[58] Shevach EM. From vanilla to 28 flavors: multiple varieties of T regulatory cells. *Immunity*. 2006 Aug;25(2):195-201.

[59] Shevach EM. Immunology. Regulating suppression. *Science (New York, NY*. 2008 Oct 10;322(5899):202-3.

[60] Shevach EM, DiPaolo RA, Andersson J, Zhao DM, Stephens GL, Thornton AM. The lifestyle of naturally occurring CD4+ CD25+ Foxp3+ regulatory T cells. *Immunol. Rev*. 2006 Aug;212:60-73.

[61] Stephens GL, Shevach EM. Foxp3+ regulatory T cells: selfishness under scrutiny. *Immunity*. 2007 Sep;27(3):417-9.

[62] Stummvoll GH, DiPaolo RJ, Huter EN, Davidson TS, Glass D, Ward JM, et al. Th1, Th2, and Th17 effector T cell-induced autoimmune gastritis differs in pathological pattern and in susceptibility to suppression by regulatory T cells. *J. Immunol*. 2008 Aug 1;181(3): 1908-16.

[63] Sakaguchi S. Regulatory T cells in the past and for the future. *Eur. J. Immunol*. 2008 Apr;38(4):901-37.

[64] Sakaguchi S, Yamaguchi T, Nomura T, Ono M. Regulatory T cells and immune tolerance. *Cell*. 2008 May 30;133(5):775-87.
[65] Belkaid Y. Regulatory T cells and infection: a dangerous necessity. *Nat. Rev. Immunol*. 2007 Nov;7(11):875-88.
[66] Shevach EM. Mechanisms of foxp3+ T regulatory cell-mediated suppression. *Immunity*. 2009 May;30(5):636-45.
[67] Garlet GP, Cardoso CR, Mariano FS, Claudino M, de Assis GF, Campanelli AP, et al. Regulatory T cells attenuate experimental periodontitis progression in mice. *Journal of clinical periodontology*. 2010 Jul;37(7):591-600.
[68] Belkaid Y. Paradoxical roles of Foxp3+ T cells during infection: from regulators to regulators. *Cell host and microbe*. 2008 Jun 12;3(6):341-3.
[69] Belkaid Y. Role of Foxp3-positive regulatory T cells during infection. *Eur. J. Immunol*. 2008 Apr;38(4):918-21.
[70] Chabaud M, Durand JM, Buchs N, Fossiez F, Page G, Frappart L, et al. Human interleukin-17: A T cell-derived proinflammatory cytokine produced by the rheumatoid synovium. *Arthritis Rheum*. 1999 May; 42(5):963-70.
[71] Braun RK, Ferrick C, Neubauer P, Sjoding M, Sterner-Kock A, Kock M, et al. IL-17 Producing gammadelta T Cells are Required for a Controlled Inflammatory Response after Bleomycin-induced Lung Injury. *Inflammation*. 2008 Mar 13.
[72] Sato K. Th17 cells and rheumatoid arthritis--from the standpoint of osteoclast differentiation. *Allergol. Int*. 2008 Jun;57(2):109-14.
[73] Aranami T, Yamamura T. Th17 Cells and autoimmune encephalomyelitis (EAE/MS). *Allergol. Int*. 2008 Jun;57(2):115-20.
[74] Kotake S, Udagawa N, Takahashi N, Matsuzaki K, Itoh K, Ishiyama S, et al. IL-17 in synovial fluids from patients with rheumatoid arthritis is a potent stimulator of osteoclastogenesis. *The Journal of clinical investigation*. 1999 May;103(9):1345-52.
[75] Beklen A, Ainola M, Hukkanen M, Gurgan C, Sorsa T, Konttinen YT. MMPs, IL-1, and TNF are regulated by IL-17 in periodontitis. *Journal of dental research*. 2007 Apr;86(4):347-51.
[76] Sato K, Suematsu A, Okamoto K, Yamaguchi A, Morishita Y, Kadono Y, et al. Th17 functions as an osteoclastogenic helper T cell subset that links T cell activation and bone destruction. *J. Exp. Med*. 2006 Nov 27;203(12):2673-82.
[77] Colic M, Vasilijic S, Gazivoda D, Vucevic D, Marjanovic M, Lukic A. Interleukin-17 plays a role in exacerbation of inflammation within

chronic periapical lesions. *European journal of oral sciences*. 2007 Aug;115(4):315-20.

[78] Vernal R, Dutzan N, Chaparro A, Puente J, Antonieta Valenzuela M, Gamonal J. Levels of interleukin-17 in gingival crevicular fluid and in supernatants of cellular cultures of gingival tissue from patients with chronic periodontitis. *Journal of clinical periodontology*. 2005 Apr;32(4):383-9.

[79] Laine ML, Loos BG, Crielaard W. Gene polymorphisms in chronic periodontitis. *International journal of dentistry*. 2010;2010:324719.

[80] Loos BG, John RP, Laine ML. Identification of genetic risk factors for periodontitis and possible mechanisms of action. *Journal of clinical periodontology*. 2005;32 Suppl 6:159-79.

[81] Stabholz A, Soskolne WA, Shapira L. Genetic and environmental risk factors for chronic periodontitis and aggressive periodontitis. *Periodontology 2000*. 2010 Jun; 53:138-53.

[82] Kinane DF, Shiba H, Hart TC. The genetic basis of periodontitis. *Periodontology 2000*. 2005;39:91-117.

[83] Yoshie H, Kobayashi T, Tai H, Galicia JC. The role of genetic polymorphisms in periodontitis. *Periodontology 2000*. 2007;43:102-32.

[84] Burns E, Bachrach G, Shapira L, Nussbaum G. Cutting Edge: TLR2 is required for the innate response to Porphyromonas gingivalis: activation leads to bacterial persistence and TLR2 deficiency attenuates induced alveolar bone resorption. *J. Immunol*. 2006 Dec 15;177(12):8296-300.

[85] Araujo LM, Ribeiro OG, Siqueira M, De Franco M, Starobinas N, Massa S, et al. Innate resistance to infection by intracellular bacterial pathogens differs in mice selected for maximal or minimal acute inflammatory response. *Eur. J. Immunol*. 1998 Sep;28(9): 2913-20.

[86] Carneiro AS, Ribeiro OG, De Franco M, Cabrera WH, Vorraro F, Siqueira M, et al. Local inflammatory reaction induced by Bothrops jararaca venom differs in mice selected for acute inflammatory response. *Toxicon*. 2002 Nov;40(11):1571-9.

[87] Ibanez OM, Stiffel C, Ribeiro OG, Cabrera WK, Massa S, de Franco M, et al. Genetics of nonspecific immunity: I. Bidirectional selective breeding of lines of mice endowed with maximal or minimal inflammatory responsiveness. *Eur. J. Immunol*. 1992 Oct; 22(10): 2555-63.

[88] Peters LC, Jensen JR, Borrego A, Cabrera WH, Baker N, Starobinas N, et al. Slc11a1 (formerly NRAMP1) gene modulates both acute

inflammatory reactions and pristane-induced arthritis in mice. *Genes and immunity*. 2007 Jan;8(1):51-6.
[89] Vigar ND, Cabrera WH, Araujo LM, Ribeiro OG, Ogata TR, Siqueira M, et al. Pristane-induced arthritis in mice selected for maximal or minimal acute inflammatory reaction. *Eur. J. Immunol.* 2000 Feb;30(2):431-7.
[90] Trombone AP, Ferreira SB, Jr., Raimundo FM, de Moura KC, Avila-Campos MJ, Silva JS, et al. Experimental periodontitis in mice selected for maximal or minimal inflammatory reactions: increased inflammatory immune responsiveness drives increased alveolar bone loss without enhancing the control of periodontal infection. *Journal of periodontal research*. 2009 Aug;44(4):443-51.
[91] Miley DD, Baumgartner MH, Cheverud JM, Roseman CC, Rogers J, McLeod DE, et al. Heritability of Alveolar Bone Loss From Periodontal Disease in a Baboon Population. A Pilot Study. *Journal of periodontology*. 2010 Nov 2.
[92] Mucci LA, Bjorkman L, Douglass CW, Pedersen NL. Environmental and heritable factors in the etiology of oral diseases--a population-based study of Swedish twins. *Journal of dental research*. 2005 Sep;84(9): 800-5.
[93] Abraham LJ, Kroeger KM. Impact of the -308 TNF promoter polymorphism on the transcriptional regulation of the TNF gene: relevance to disease. *J. Leukoc. Biol.* 1999 Oct;66(4):562-6.
[94] Kroeger KM, Steer JH, Joyce DA, Abraham LJ. Effects of stimulus and cell type on the expression of the -308 tumour necrosis factor promoter polymorphism. *Cytokine*. 2000 Feb;12(2):110-9.
[95] Gao J, Shan G, Sun B, Thompson PJ, Gao X. Association between polymorphism of tumour necrosis factor alpha-308 gene promoter and asthma: a meta-analysis. *Thorax*. 2006 Jun;61(6):466-71.
[96] Lee YH, Ji JD, Song GG. Tumor necrosis factor-alpha promoter -308 A/G polymorphism and rheumatoid arthritis susceptibility: a metaanalysis. *The Journal of rheumatology*. 2007 Jan;34(1):43-9.
[97] Zhang J, Dou C, Song Y, Ji C, Gu S, Xie Y, et al. Polymorphisms of tumor necrosis factor-alpha are associated with increased susceptibility to gastric cancer: a meta-analysis. *Journal of human genetics*. 2008 Mar 19.
[98] Galbraith GM, Steed RB, Sanders JJ, Pandey JP. Tumor necrosis factor alpha production by oral leukocytes: influence of tumor necrosis factor genotype. *Journal of periodontology*. 1998 Apr;69(4):428-33.

[99] Galbraith GM, Hendley TM, Sanders JJ, Palesch Y, Pandey JP. Polymorphic cytokine genotypes as markers of disease severity in adult periodontitis. *Journal of clinical periodontology*. 1999 Nov;26(11): 705-9.

[100] Huynh-Ba G, Lang NP, Tonetti MS, Salvi GE. The association of the composite IL-1 genotype with periodontitis progression and/or treatment outcomes: a systematic review. *Journal of clinical periodontology*. 2007 Apr;34(4):305-17.

[101] Shapira L, Wilensky A, Kinane DF. Effect of genetic variability on the inflammatory response to periodontal infection. *Journal of clinical periodontology*. 2005;32 Suppl 6:72-86.

[102] Zondervan KT, Cardon LR, Kennedy SH. What makes a good case-control study? Design issues for complex traits such as endometriosis. *Human reproduction (Oxford, England)*. 2002 Jun;17(6):1415-23.

[103] Page RC, Beck JD. Risk assessment for periodontal diseases. *International dental journal*. 1997 Apr;47(2):61-87.

[104] Kornman KS, Crane A, Wang HY, di Giovine FS, Newman MG, Pirk FW, et al. The interleukin-1 genotype as a severity factor in adult periodontal disease. *Journal of clinical periodontology*. 1997 Jan; 24(1):72-7.

[105] Shapira L, Stabholz A, Rieckmann P, Kruse N. Genetic polymorphism of the tumor necrosis factor (TNF)-alpha promoter region in families with localized early-onset periodontitis. *Journal of periodontal research*. 2001 Jun;36(3):183-6.

[106] Nikolopoulos GK, Dimou NL, Hamodrakas SJ, Bagos PG. Cytokine gene polymorphisms in periodontal disease: a meta-analysis of 53 studies including 4178 cases and 4590 controls. *Journal of clinical periodontology*. 2008 Sep;35(9):754-67.

[107] Garlet GP, Trombone AP, Menezes R, Letra A, Repeke CE, Vieira AE, et al. The use of chronic gingivitis as reference status increases the power and odds of periodontitis genetic studies - a proposal based in the exposure concept and clearer resistance and susceptibility phenotypes definition. *Journal of clinical periodontology*. 2012 Jan 30.

[108] Edwards BJ, Haynes C, Levenstien MA, Finch SJ, Gordon D. Power and sample size calculations in the presence of phenotype errors for case/control genetic association studies. *BMC Genet*. 2005;6:18.

[109] Wojczynski MK, Tiwari HK. Definition of phenotype. *Adv. Genet.* 2008;60:75-105.

[110] Day N. Commentary: How small is small? *International journal of epidemiology*. 2009 Feb;38(1):274-5.

[111] Burton PR, Hansell AL, Fortier I, Manolio TA, Khoury MJ, Little J, et al. Size matters: just how big is BIG?: Quantifying realistic sample size requirements for human genome epidemiology. *International journal of epidemiology*. 2009 Feb;38(1):263-73.

[112] Schafer AS, Jepsen S, Loos BG. Periodontal genetics: a decade of genetic association studies mandates better study designs. *Journal of clinical periodontology*. 2011 Feb;38(2):103-7.

[113] Zondervan KT, Cardon LR. Designing candidate gene and genome-wide case-control association studies. *Nature protocols*. 2007;2(10):2492-501.

[114] Buyske S, Yang G, Matise TC, Gordon D. When a case is not a case: effects of phenotype misclassification on power and sample size requirements for the transmission disequilibrium test with affected child trios. *Human heredity*. 2009; 67(4):287-92.

[115] Evangelou E, Fellay J, Colombo S, Martinez-Picado J, Obel N, Goldstein DB, et al. Impact of phenotype definition on genome-wide association signals: empirical evaluation in human immunodeficiency virus type 1 infection. *Am. J. Epidemiol*. 2011 Jun 1;173(11):1336-42.

[116] Ozturk A, Vieira AR. TLR4 as a risk factor for periodontal disease: a reappraisal. *Journal of clinical periodontology*. 2009 Apr;36(4):279-86.

[117] Garlet GP, Cardoso CR, Campanelli AP, Martins W, Jr., Silva JS. Expression of suppressors of cytokine signaling in diseased periodontal tissues: a stop signal for disease progression? *Journal of periodontal research*. 2006 Dec;41(6):580-4.

[118] Sanz M, van Winkelhoff AJ. Periodontal infections: understanding the complexity--consensus of the Seventh European Workshop on Periodontology. *Journal of clinical periodontology*. 2011 Mar;38 Suppl 11:3-6.

[119] Kadowaki T, Nakayama K, Okamoto K, Abe N, Baba A, Shi Y, et al. Porphyromonas gingivalis proteinases as virulence determinants in progression of periodontal diseases. *Journal of biochemistry*. 2000 Aug;128(2):153-9.

[120] Lamont RJ, Jenkinson HF. Life below the gum line: pathogenic mechanisms of Porphyromonas gingivalis. *Microbiol. Mol. Biol. Rev*. 1998 Dec;62(4):1244-63.

[121] Silva N, Dutzan N, Hernandez M, Dezerega A, Rivera O, Aguillon JC, et al. Characterization of progressive periodontal lesions in chronic periodontitis patients: levels of chemokines, cytokines, matrix

metalloproteinase-13, periodontal pathogens and inflammatory cells. *Journal of clinical periodontology*. 2008 Mar;35(3):206-14.

[122] Kowalski J, Gorska R, Dragan M, Kozak I. Clinical state of the patients with periodontitis, IL-1 polymorphism and pathogens in periodontal pocket--is there a link? (An introductory report). *Advances in medical sciences*. 2006;51 Suppl 1:9-12.

[123] Bodet C, Chandad F, Grenier D. Inflammatory responses of a macrophage/epithelial cell co-culture model to mono and mixed infections with Porphyromonas gingivalis, Treponema denticola, and Tannerella forsythia. *Microbes Infect*. 2006 Jan;8(1):27-35.

[124] Yang HW, Huang YF, Chou MY. Occurrence of Porphyromonas gingivalis and Tannerella forsythensis in periodontally diseased and healthy subjects. *Journal of periodontology*. 2004 Aug;75(8):1077-83.

[125] Kuramitsu HK, Chen W, Ikegami A. Biofilm formation by the periodontopathic bacteria Treponema denticola and Porphyromonas gingivalis. *Journal of periodontology*. 2005 Nov;76(11 Suppl):2047-51.

[126] Sharma A, Inagaki S, Sigurdson W, Kuramitsu HK. Synergy between Tannerella forsythia and Fusobacterium nucleatum in biofilm formation. *Oral Microbiol Immunol*. 2005 Feb;20(1):39-42.

[127] Mineoka T, Awano S, Rikimaru T, Kurata H, Yoshida A, Ansai T, et al. Site-Specific Development of Periodontal Disease Is Associated With Increased Levels of Porphyromonas gingivalis, Treponema denticola, and Tannerella forsythia in Subgingival Plaque. *Journal of periodontology*. 2008 Apr;79(4):670-6.

[128] Kesavalu L, Sathishkumar S, Bakthavatchalu V, Matthews C, Dawson D, Steffen M, et al. Rat model of polymicrobial infection, immunity, and alveolar bone resorption in periodontal disease. *Infection and immunity*. 2007 Apr;75(4):1704-12.

[129] Iwata T, Mitani A, Ishihara Y, Tanaka S, Yamamoto G, Kikuchi T, et al. Actinobacillus actinomycetemcomitans Y4 capsular polysaccharide induces IL-1beta mRNA expression through the JNK pathway in differentiated THP-1 cells. *Clin. Exp. Immunol*. 2005 Aug;141(2):261-9.

[130] Kelk P, Claesson R, Hanstrom L, Lerner UH, Kalfas S, Johansson A. Abundant secretion of bioactive interleukin-1beta by human macrophages induced by Actinobacillus actinomycetemcomitans leukotoxin. *Infection and immunity*. 2005 Jan; 73(1):453-8.

[131] Ohguchi Y, Ishihara Y, Ohguchi M, Koide M, Shirozu N, Naganawa T, et al. Capsular polysaccharide from Actinobacillus actinomycetemcomitans inhibits IL-6 and IL-8 production in human

gingival fibroblast. *Journal of periodontal research*. 2003 Apr; 38(2): 191-7.

[132] Kurita-Ochiai T, Ochiai K. Immunosuppressive factor from Actinobacillus actinomycetemcomitans down regulates cytokine production. *Infection and immunity*. 1996 Jan;64(1):50-4.

[133] Schacher B, Baron F, Rossberg M, Wohlfeil M, Arndt R, Eickholz P. Aggregatibacter actinomycetemcomitans as indicator for aggressive periodontitis by two analysing strategies. *Journal of clinical periodontology*. 2007 Jul;34(7):566-73.

[134] Bodet C, Chandad F, Grenier D. Porphyromonas gingivalis-induced inflammatory mediator profile in an ex vivo human whole blood model. *Clin. Exp. Immunol*. 2006 Jan;143(1):50-7.

[135] Kesavalu L, Chandrasekar B, Ebersole JL. In vivo induction of proinflammatory cytokines in mouse tissue by Porphyromonas gingivalis and Actinobacillus actinomycetemcomitans. *Oral Microbiol. Immunol*. 2002 Jun;17(3):177-80.

[136] Lin YY, Huang JH, Lai YY, Huang HC, Hu SW. Tissue destruction induced by Porphyromonas gingivalis infection in a mouse chamber model is associated with host tumor necrosis factor generation. *Infection and immunity*. 2005 Dec;73(12):7946-52.

[137] Hirose K, Isogai E, Miura H, Ueda I. Levels of Porphyromonas gingivalis Fimbriae and inflammatory cytokines in gingival crevicular fluid from adult human subjects. *Microbiology and immunology*. 1997;41(1):21-6.

[138] Graves DT, Oskoui M, Volejnikova S, Naguib G, Cai S, Desta T, et al. Tumor necrosis factor modulates fibroblast apoptosis, PMN recruitment, and osteoclast formation in response to P. gingivalis infection. *Journal of dental research*. 2001 Oct;80(10):1875-9.

[139] Agarwal S, Piesco NP, Johns LP, Riccelli AE. Differential expression of IL-1 beta, TNF-alpha, IL-6, and IL-8 in human monocytes in response to lipopolysaccharides from different microbes. *Journal of dental research*. 1995 Apr;74(4):1057-65.

[140] Kurita-Ochiai T, Ochiai K, Saito N, Ikeda T. Adoptive transfer of suppressor T cells induced by Actinobacillus actinomycetemcomitans regulates immune response. *Journal of periodontal research*. 1994 Jan;29(1):1-8.

[141] Rabie GH. Induction of fungal disease resistance in Vicia faba by dual inoculation with Rhizobium leguminosarum and vesicular-arbuscular mycorrhizal fungi. *Mycopathologia*. 1998;141(3):159-66.

[142] Tanabe SI, Grenier D. Macrophage tolerance response to Aggregatibacter actinomycetemcomitans lipopolysaccharide induces differential regulation of tumor necrosis factor-alpha, interleukin-1 beta and matrix metalloproteinase 9 secretion. *Journal of periodontal research*. 2008 Jun;43(3):372-7.

[143] Fernandes KP, Mayer MP, Ando ES, Ulbrich AG, Amarente-Mendes JG, Russo M. Inhibition of interferon-gamma-induced nitric oxide production in endotoxin-activated macrophages by cytolethal distending toxin. *Oral Microbiol. Immunol.* 2008 Oct; 23(5):360-6.

[144] Slots J. Herpesviral-bacterial synergy in the pathogenesis of human periodontitis. *Current opinion in infectious diseases*. 2007 Jun;20(3): 278-83.

[145] Cappuyns I, Gugerli P, Mombelli A. Viruses in periodontal disease - a review. *Oral diseases*. 2005 Jul;11(4):219-29.

[146] Saygun I, Kubar A, Sahin S, Sener K, Slots J. Quantitative analysis of association between herpesviruses and bacterial pathogens in periodontitis. *Journal of periodontal research*. 2008 Jun;43(3):352-9.

[147] Wara-Aswapati N, Boch JA, Auron PE. Activation of interleukin 1beta gene transcription by human cytomegalovirus: molecular mechanisms and relevance to periodontitis. *Oral Microbiol. Immunol.* 2003 Apr;18(2):67-71.

[148] Yin MT, Dobkin JF, Grbic JT. Epidemiology, pathogenesis, and management of human immunodeficiency virus infection in patients with periodontal disease. *Periodontology 2000*. 2007;44:55-81.

[149] Caskey MF, Morgan DJ, Porto AF, Giozza SP, Muniz AL, Orge GO, et al. Clinical manifestations associated with HTLV type I infection: a cross-sectional study. *AIDS research and human retroviruses*. 2007 Mar;23(3):365-71.

[150] Giozza SP, Santos SB, Martinelli M, Porto MA, Muniz AL, Carvalho EM. [Salivary and lacrymal gland disorders and HTLV-1 infection]. *Revue de stomatologie et de chirurgie maxillo-faciale*. 2008 Jun;109(3):153-7.

[151] Garlet GP, Giozza SP, Silveira EM, Claudino M, Santos SB, Avila-Campos MJ, et al. Association of human T lymphotropic virus 1 amplification of periodontitis severity with altered cytokine expression in response to a standard periodontopathogen infection. *Clin. Infect. Dis.* 2010 Feb 1;50(3):e11-8.

[152] Goncalves DU, Proietti FA, Barbosa-Stancioli EF, Martins ML, Ribas JG, Martins-Filho OA, et al. HTLV-1-associated myelopathy/tropical

spastic paraparesis (HAM/TSP) inflammatory network. *Inflammation and allergy drug targets*. 2008 Jun; 7(2):98-107.
[153] Yamano Y, Takenouchi N, Li HC, Tomaru U, Yao K, Grant CW, et al. Virus-induced dysfunction of CD4+CD25+ T cells in patients with HTLV-I-associated neuroimmunological disease. *The Journal of clinical investigation*. 2005 May; 115(5):1361-8.
[154] Grant C, Oh U, Yao K, Yamano Y, Jacobson S. Dysregulation of TGF-beta signaling and regulatory and effector T-cell function in virus-induced neuroinflammatory disease. *Blood*. 2008 Jun 15;111(12): 5601-9.
[155] Michaelsson J, Barbosa HM, Jordan KA, Chapman JM, Brunialti MK, Neto WK, et al. The frequency of CD127low expressing CD4+CD25high T regulatory cells is inversely correlated with human T lymphotrophic virus type-1 (HTLV-1) proviral load in HTLV-1-infection and HTLV-1-associated myelopathy/tropical spastic paraparesis. *BMC immunology*. 2008;9:41.
[156] Lee JE, Choi JH, Lee JH, Lee MG. Gene SNPs and mutations in clinical genetic testing: haplotype-based testing and analysis. *Mutation research*. 2005 Jun 3;573(1-2):195-204.
[157] Zintzaras E, Lau J. Synthesis of genetic association studies for pertinent gene-disease associations requires appropriate methodological and statistical approaches. *Journal of clinical epidemiology*. 2008 Jul;61(7):634-45.
[158] Lettre G, Rioux JD. Autoimmune diseases: insights from genome-wide association studies. *Human molecular genetics*. 2008 Oct 15;17(R2):R116-21.
[159] Zhernakova A, van Diemen CC, Wijmenga C. Detecting shared pathogenesis from the shared genetics of immune-related diseases. *Nat Rev Genet*. 2009 Jan;10(1):43-55.
[160] Somers EC, Thomas SL, Smeeth L, Hall AJ. Autoimmune diseases co-occurring within individuals and within families: a systematic review. *Epidemiology (Cambridge, Mass*. 2006 Mar;17(2):202-17.
[161] Pischon N, Pischon T, Kroger J, Gulmez E, Kleber BM, Bernimoulin JP, et al. Association among rheumatoid arthritis, oral hygiene, and periodontitis. *Journal of periodontology*. 2008 Jun;79(6):979-86.
[162] Kasser UR, Gleissner C, Dehne F, Michel A, Willershausen-Zonnchen B, Bolten WW. Risk for periodontal disease in patients with longstanding rheumatoid arthritis. *Arthritis Rheum*. 1997 Dec;40(12): 2248-51.

[163] Mercado FB, Marshall RI, Klestov AC, Bartold PM. Relationship between rheumatoid arthritis and periodontitis. *Journal of periodontology*. 2001 Jun;72(6):779-87.

[164] Nilsson M, Kopp S. Gingivitis and periodontitis are related to repeated high levels of circulating tumor necrosis factor-alpha in patients with rheumatoid arthritis. *Journal of periodontology*. 2008 Sep;79(9): 1689-96.

[165] Bartold PM, Marshall RI, Haynes DR. Periodontitis and rheumatoid arthritis: a review. *Journal of periodontology*. 2005 Nov;76(11 Suppl):2066-74.

[166] de Pablo P, Chapple IL, Buckley CD, Dietrich T. Periodontitis in systemic rheumatic diseases. *Nat. Rev. Rheumatol.* 2009 Apr;5(4): 218-24.

[167] de Pablo P, Dietrich T, McAlindon TE. Association of periodontal disease and tooth loss with rheumatoid arthritis in the US population. *The Journal of rheumatology*. 2008 Jan;35(1):70-6.

[168] McInnes IB, Schett G. Cytokines in the pathogenesis of rheumatoid arthritis. *Nat. Rev. Immunol.* 2007 Jun;7(6):429-42.

[169] Golub LM, Payne JB, Reinhardt RA, Nieman G. Can systemic diseases co-induce (not just exacerbate) periodontitis? A hypothetical "two-hit" model. *Journal of dental research*. 2006 Feb;85(2):102-5.

[170] Garlet GP, Cardoso CR, Campanelli AP, Garlet TP, Avila-Campos MJ, Cunha FQ, et al. The essential role of IFN-gamma in the control of lethal Aggregatibacter actinomycetemcomitans infection in mice. *Microbes Infect.* 2008 Apr;10(5):489-96.

[171] Ortiz P, Bissada NF, Palomo L, Han YW, Al-Zahrani MS, Panneerselvam A, et al. Periodontal therapy reduces the severity of active rheumatoid arthritis in patients treated with or without tumor necrosis factor inhibitors. *Journal of periodontology*. 2009 Apr; 80(4):535-40.

[172] Al-Katma MK, Bissada NF, Bordeaux JM, Sue J, Askari AD. Control of periodontal infection reduces the severity of active rheumatoid arthritis. *J. Clin. Rheumatol.* 2007 Jun;13(3):134-7.

[173] Miranda LA, Islabao AG, Fischer RG, Figueredo CM, Oppermann RV, Gustafsson A. Decreased interleukin-1beta and elastase in the gingival crevicular fluid of individuals undergoing anti-inflammatory treatment for rheumatoid arthritis. *Journal of periodontology*. 2007 Aug;78(8): 1612-9.

[174] Rosenstein ED, Greenwald RA, Kushner LJ, Weissmann G. Hypothesis: the humoral immune response to oral bacteria provides a stimulus for the development of rheumatoid arthritis. *Inflammation*. 2004 Dec;28(6): 311-8.

[175] Queiroz-Junior CM, Madeira MF, Coelho FM, Costa VV, Bessoni RL, Sousa LF, et al. Experimental arthritis triggers periodontal disease in mice: involvement of TNF-alpha and the oral Microbiota. *J. Immunol*. 2011 Oct 1;187(7):3821-30.

[176] Trombone AP, Claudino M, Colavite P, de Assis GF, Avila-Campos MJ, Silva JS, et al. Periodontitis and arthritis interaction in mice involves a shared hyper-inflammatory genotype and functional immunological interferences. *Genes and immunity*. 2010 Apr 29.

[177] Ramamurthy NS, Greenwald RA, Celiker MY, Shi EY. Experimental arthritis in rats induces biomarkers of periodontitis which are ameliorated by gene therapy with tissue inhibitor of matrix metalloproteinases. *Journal of periodontology*. 2005 Feb;76(2):229-33.

[178] Biyikoglu B, Buduneli N, Kardesler L, Aksu K, Oder G, Kutukculer N. Evaluation of t-PA, PAI-2, IL-1beta and PGE(2) in gingival crevicular fluid of rheumatoid arthritis patients with periodontal disease. *Journal of clinical periodontology*. 2006 Sep; 33(9):605-11.

[179] Yoshida A, Nakano Y, Yamashita Y, Oho T, Ito H, Kondo M, et al. Immunodominant region of Actinobacillus actinomycetemcomitans 40-kilodalton heat shock protein in patients with rheumatoid arthritis. *Journal of dental research*. 2001 Jan;80(1):346-50.

[180] The J, Ebersole JL. Rheumatoid factor from periodontitis patients cross-reacts with epitopes on oral bacteria. *Oral diseases*. 1996 Dec;2(4): 253-62.

[181] Ogrendik M, Kokino S, Ozdemir F, Bird PS, Hamlet S. Serum antibodies to oral anaerobic bacteria in patients with rheumatoid arthritis. *MedGenMed*. 2005;7(2):2.

[182] Liao F, Li Z, Wang Y, Shi B, Gong Z, Cheng X. Porphyromonasgingivalis may play an important role in the pathogenesis of periodontitis-associated rheumatoid arthritis. *Medical hypotheses*. 2009 Jun;72(6):732-5.

[183] Moen K, Brun JG, Valen M, Skartveit L, Eribe EK, Olsen I, et al. Synovial inflammation in active rheumatoid arthritis and psoriatic arthritis facilitates trapping of a variety of oral bacterial DNAs. *Clinical and experimental rheumatology*. 2006 Nov-Dec;24(6):656-63.

[184] Moen K, Bertelsen LT, Hellem S, Jonsson R, Brun JG. Salivary gland and temporomandibular joint involvement in rheumatoid arthritis: relation to disease activity. *Oral diseases*. 2005 Jan;11(1):27-34.

[185] Moen K, Brun JG, Madland TM, Tynning T, Jonsson R. Immunoglobulin G and A antibody responses to Bacteroides forsythus and Prevotella intermedia in sera and synovial fluids of arthritis patients. *Clinical and diagnostic laboratory immunology*. 2003 Nov;10(6): 1043-50.

[186] Rantapaa-Dahlqvist S, de Jong BA, Berglin E, Hallmans G, Wadell G, Stenlund H, et al. Antibodies against cyclic citrullinated peptide and IgA rheumatoid factor predict the development of rheumatoid arthritis. *Arthritis Rheum*. 2003 Oct;48(10):2741-9.

[187] Agrawal S, Misra R, Aggarwal A. Autoantibodies in rheumatoid arthritis: association with severity of disease in established RA. *Clin Rheumatol*. 2007 Feb;26(2):201-4.

[188] Wegner N, Wait R, Sroka A, Eick S, Nguyen KA, Lundberg K, et al. Peptidylarginine deiminase from Porphyromonas gingivalis citrullinates human fibrinogen and alpha-enolase: implications for autoimmunity in rheumatoid arthritis. *Arthritis Rheum*. 2010 Sep;62(9):2662-72.

[189] Claudino M, Ceolin DS, Alberti S, Cestari TM, Spadella CT, Rubira-Bullen IR, et al. Alloxan-induced diabetes triggers the development of periodontal disease in rats. *PloS one*. 2007;2(12):e1320.

[190] Standards of medical care in diabetes--2011. *Diabetes care*. 2011 Jan;34 Suppl 1:S11-61.

[191] Lalla E, Papapanou PN. Diabetes mellitus and periodontitis: a tale of two common interrelated diseases. *Nat. Rev. Endocrinol*. 2011 Dec;7(12):738-48.

[192] Lamster IB, Lalla E, Borgnakke WS, Taylor GW. The relationship between oral health and diabetes mellitus. *Journal of the American Dental Association (1939)*. 2008 Oct;139 Suppl:19S-24S.

[193] Ramasamy R, Yan SF, Schmidt AM. Receptor for AGE (RAGE): signaling mechanisms in the pathogenesis of diabetes and its complications. *Annals of the New York Academy of Sciences*. 2011 Dec; 1243(1):88-102.

[194] Barlovic DP, Soro-Paavonen A, Jandeleit-Dahm KA. RAGE biology, atherosclerosis and diabetes. *Clin. Sci. (Lond)*. 2011 Jul;121(2):43-55.

[195] Lalla E, Lamster IB, Feit M, Huang L, Spessot A, Qu W, et al. Blockade of RAGE suppresses periodontitis-associated bone loss in diabetic mice. *The Journal of clinical investigation*. 2000 Apr;105(8):1117-24.

[196] Sima C, Rhourida K, Van Dyke TE, Gyurko R. Type 1 diabetes predisposes to enhanced gingival leukocyte margination and macromolecule extravasation in vivo. *Journal of periodontal research*. 2010 Dec;45(6):748-56.

[197] Shetty N, Thomas B, Ramesh A. Comparison of neutrophil functions in diabetic and healthy subjects with chronic generalized periodontitis. *J. Indian Soc. Periodontol*. 2008 May;12(2):41-4.

[198] Arbes SJ, Jr., Sever ML, Vaughn B, Cohen EA, Zeldin DC. Oral pathogens and allergic disease: results from the Third National Health and Nutrition Examination Survey. *J. Allergy Clin. Immunol*. 2006 Nov;118(5):1169-75.

[199] Friedrich N, Kocher T, Wallaschofski H, Schwahn C, Ludemann J, Kerner W, et al. Inverse association between periodontitis and respiratory allergies in patients with type 1 diabetes mellitus. *Journal of clinical periodontology*. 2008 Apr;35(4):305-10.

[200] Strachan DP. Hay fever, hygiene, and household size. *BMJ (Clinical research ed*. 1989 Nov 18;299(6710):1259-60.

[201] Okada H, Kuhn C, Feillet H, Bach JF. The 'hygiene hypothesis' for autoimmune and allergic diseases: an update. *Clin. Exp. Immunol*. Apr;160(1):1-9.

[202] Card JW, Carey MA, Voltz JW, Bradbury JA, Ferguson CD, Cohen EA, et al. Modulation of allergic airway inflammation by the oral pathogen Porphyromonas gingivalis. *Infection and immunity*. 2010 Jun;78(6):2488-96.

[203] da Fonseca DM, Trombone AP, Repeke CE, Avila-Campos MJ, Coelho-Castelo AA, Silva JS, et al. Functional interferences in host inflammatory immune response by airway allergic inflammation restrain experimental periodontitis development in mice. *Journal of clinical periodontology*. 2011 Feb;38(2):131-41.

[204] Appay V, van Lier RA, Sallusto F, Roederer M. Phenotype and function of human T lymphocyte subsets: consensus and issues. *Cytometry A*. 2008 Nov;73(11):975-83.

[205] Jarnicki AG, Fallon PG. T helper type-2 cytokine responses: potential therapeutic targets. *Current opinion in pharmacology*. 2003 Aug;3(4):449-55.

[206] Agnello D, Lankford CS, Bream J, Morinobu A, Gadina M, O'Shea JJ, et al. Cytokines and transcription factors that regulate T helper cell differentiation: new players and new insights. *Journal of clinical immunology*. 2003 May;23(3):147-61.

[207] Bluestone JA, Mackay CR, O'Shea JJ, Stockinger B. The functional plasticity of T cell subsets. *Nat. Rev. Immunol.* 2009 Nov;9(11):811-6.

[208] Newcomb DC, Zhou W, Moore ML, Goleniewska K, Hershey GK, Kolls JK, et al. A functional IL-13 receptor is expressed on polarized murine CD4+ Th17 cells and IL-13 signaling attenuates Th17 cytokine production. *J. Immunol.* 2009 May 1;182(9): 5317-21.

[209] Saidenberg-Kermanac'h N, Bessis N, Lemeiter D, de Vernejoul MC, Boissier MC, Cohen-Solal M. Interleukin-4 cellular gene therapy and osteoprotegerin decrease inflammation-associated bone resorption in collagen-induced arthritis. *Journal of clinical immunology*. 2004 Jul;24(4):370-8.

[210] Ihn H, Yamane K, Asano Y, Kubo M, Tamaki K. IL-4 up-regulates the expression of tissue inhibitor of metalloproteinase-2 in dermal fibroblasts via the p38 mitogen-activated protein kinase dependent pathway. *J. Immunol.* 2002 Feb 15;168(4):1895-902.

[211] Giannopoulou C, Kamma JJ, Mombelli A. Effect of inflammation, smoking and stress on gingival crevicular fluid cytokine level. *Journal of clinical periodontology*. 2003 Feb;30(2):145-53.

[212] Osada Y, Shimizu S, Kumagai T, Yamada S, Kanazawa T. Schistosoma mansoni infection reduces severity of collagen-induced arthritis via down-regulation of pro-inflammatory mediators. *International journal for parasitology*. 2009 Mar;39(4): 457-64.

[213] Garlet GP. Destructive and protective roles of cytokines in periodontitis: host defense and tissue destruction viewpoints. *Journal of dental research*. 2010;in press.

In: Bone Loss
Editor: Kuo-Cheng Lu
ISBN: 978-1-62417-169-7

Chapter 7

DIETARY GREEN TEA EXTRACT AND VITAMIN D INCREASED BONE MINERAL DENSITY IN ELDERLY WOMEN IN ISHIKAWA PREFECTURE, JAPAN

***Noboru Hasegawa*[1] *and Miyako Mochizuki*[2]**
[1]Department of Health and Medical Sciences, Ishikawa Prefectural Nursing University, Kahoku City, Ishikawa, Japan
[2]Higashiosaka Junior College, Higashiosaka, Japan

ABSTRACT

Green tea, a traditional oriental beverage, has dietary antioxidant components, but little is known about its role in the bone health of elderly women. Vitamin D deficiency in adults can exacerbate osteopenia and osteoporosis. We studied the protective effect of green tea extract and vitamin D on bone mineral density (BMD) in elderly women in Ishikawa Prefecture, Japan. Our double-blind, randomized controlled trial (5 months) included healthy postmenopausal elderly women (72.5 ± 4.7 years of age, mean ± SD). Treatment groups consisted of a placebo control group (5.85 μg/day vitamin D, n=24) and a green tea group (360 mg/day green tea extract and 5.85 μg/day vitamin D, n=30). BMD of the right heel was measured by bone ultrasound of T scores were assessed. The green tea group had a statistically significant smaller reduction in T scores ($p<0.01$) compared to the placebo group ($p<0.05$). These results suggest that green tea extract increases BMD in elderly women. Green tea contains several polyphenolic components, and (−) epigallocatechin gallate (EGCG) is its most abundant catechin. Using ovariectomy (OVX), we studied the protective effect of EGCG on the mechanical properties of femur bone strength loss in estrogen-deprived middle-aged rats. OVX significantly decreased femur bone strength measured by the three-point bending test, and EGCG (16 mg/kg was administered daily by gavage for 3 months) suppressed bone loss induced by OVX. To investigate the action EGCG has on bone formation, we studied its effect on mineralization and estrogen receptor expression in osteoblastic MC3T3-E1 cells. Calcium depositions by alizarin red S staining and estrogen receptor β (ERβ) were increased after culture with EGCG (10 μg /mL). These observations confirmed that green tea extract can increase BMD via osteoblast activation in elderly women.

INTRODUCTION

Osteoporosis is a degenerative bone disease characterized by low bone mass and microarchitectural detereioration of bone tissue [1]. In Japan, osteoporosis is also a major public health problem that affects a large number of elderly people. Osteoporosis associated with estrogen deficiency is the most common cause of age-related bone loss. Lifestyle issues including diet and physical activity are important modifiable factors in the development and maintenance of bone mass [2]. Also, total intake of calcium and other nutrients such as vitamin D are effective in preventing bone loss [3]. It is known that the bone is maintained by bone formation by osteoblasts and bone resorption by osteoclasts. An imbalance between bone formation and bone resorption leads to metabolic bone diseases. In the past few years, the protective effects of antioxidative flavonoids in fruits and vegetables against osteoporosis have been reported [4]. It is well known that green tea (Camellia sinensis) is a traditional beverage in Japan and much of Asia. Several biological properties containing antimicrobial, antioxidative, antimutagenic, and anticarcinogenic activities were reported. Green tea contains several polyphenolic compounds including (-) epigallocatechin gallate (EGCG), (-) epicatechin gallate, (-) epicatechin, and (-) epigallocatechin [5]. EGCG is an important constituent of green tea, and is known to possess strong biological activity through its antioxidative strengths. In the animal study, green tea polyphenol supplementation attenuated bone loss in aged orchidectomized [6] and middle-aged female rats [7]. Epidemiological evidence has shown an association between tea consumption and the prevention of bone loss in the elderly population [8, 9, 10]. We studied the protective effect of a dietary supplement of green tea extract (GTE) and vitamin D on bone mineral density (BMD) in elderly women of Ishikawa Prefecture, Japan. We also studied the effect of EGCG on BMD in multiparous ovariectomized rats and on the mineralization of osteoblast-like MC3T3-E1 cells.

Materials and Methods

Subjects

Prior to the study, approval was obtained from the ethics committee of Ishikawa Prefectural University (project registration number: 332-2). The study was conducted with women over 65 years of age residing in Kahoku City, Ishikawa Prefecture, Japan. After obtaining informed consent, we enrolled 54 Japanese women in this study.

Study Design

Our double-blind, randomized controlled trial (5 months) included healthy postmenopausal elderly women (72.5 ± 4.7 years of age, mean ± SD). Treatment groups consisted of a placebo control group (5.85 μg/day vitamin D, n=24) and a green tea group (360 mg/day GTE and 5.85 μg/day vitamin D, n=30). Placebo and GTE of the same lot, respectively, were purchased from Api Co., Ltd., Gifu, Japan. Each GTE tablet contained 120 mg of the GTE ingredient [more than 25% of EGCG] and 1.95 μg of vitamin D3. Placebo tablets contained 1.95 μg of vitamin D3 and were made of the same size and color as the GTE tablet. Bone mineral density (BMD) was measured using an ultrasound bone densitometer (CM-200, Furuno Electric Co., Ltd., Hyogo, Japan) over the left heel. Body composition was measured using InBody (Biospace Japan, Inc., Tokyo, Japan).

Animal Studies

Animal studies were performed according to our previous methods [11]. Eighteen female multiparous Sprague-Dawley (SD) rats weighing 350 ± 10 g were obtained from Charles River Japan, Inc. (Tokyo, Japan). The rats were housed in standard cages and fed with standard laboratory chow and tap water ad libitum. All procedures for handling animals were approved by the Animal Experimentation Committee of Gifu Women's University Graduate School of Human Life Science. Bilateral ovariectomy was performed and all the animals were killed by decapitation. The sham-operated (SHAM) rats were subjected to the same general surgical procedure as the ovariectomized (OVX) rats, except that their ovaries were not excised. EGCG (16 mg/kg, Sigma-Aldrich, St. Louis, MO, USA) was administered daily by gavage for 3 months after OVX. After killing, the femurs were subjected to a three-point bending test by a previously described method [11]. Briefly, the left femur was cleaned to remove its surrounding soft tissue and subjected to a material testing machine (EZ-test, Shimadzu, Kyoto, Japan) at a constant deformation rate of 5 mm/min with a rod at the upper midpoint of the femur. The test range was 0 to 500 N. The two outer supporting points were fixed 10 mm apart with a single central point positioned at the midpoint of the specimen. During the three-point bending test, load-deformation data was recorded and subsequently analyzed, and the maximal force (N) to break the femur was determined as bone strength.

Cellular Studies

Osteoblastic MC3T3-E1 cells (purchased from RIKEN Cell Bank, Tsukuba, Japan) were cultured at 37°C in 5% CO_2 in an α-modified minimal essential medium (α-MEM, Invitrogen, Life Technologies Corp., Carlsbad, CA, USA) supplemented with 10% fetal bovine serum (BioWest S.A.S, France), 100 U/mL penicillin, and 100 μg/mL streptomycin (Invitrogen, Life Technologies Corp., Carlsbad, CA, USA). Disodium β-glycerophosphate (10 mM, Sigma-Aldrich, St. Louis, MO, USA) and L-ascorbic acid (50 μg/mL, Sigma-Aldrich, St. Louis, MO, USA) were added to the culture medium to differentiate to osteoblasts for 28 days [12]. The calcium depositions of MC3T3-E1 cell cultures were stained by alizarin red S solution (Wako Pure Chemical Industries, Ltd., Osaka, Japan). EGCG (10 μg/mL) was added throughout the culture. Intracellular protein extracts were analyzed on a 12% polyacrylamide mini-gel electrophoresis at room temperature. After transfer onto PVDF membranes (Merck Millipore Corp., Tokyo, Japan), the membranes were blocked, incubated with a 1:500 dilution of anti-mouse estrogen receptor β polyclonal antibody (Assay Biotechnology Company Inc., Sunnyvale, CA, USA), and incubated with a 1:300 dilution of anti-rabbit IgG

(Biomedical Technologies, Inc., Stoughton, MA, USA) with SNAP i.d. (Merck Millipore Corp., Tokyo, Japan). The immunoreactive bands were detected with ECL detection reagent (WZ-ECL, Biological Industries Israel Beit-Haemek, Ltd., Israel).

Statistical Analysis

Results are expressed as the mean ± SD, and differences between before and after intervention with supplements were evaluated using the paired *t*-test. A probability value of less than 0.05 was considered to indicate statistical significance.

RESULTS AND DISCUSSION

Human Studies

Characteristics of the study participants are shown in Table 1.

Table 1. Characteristics of study participants

Variables	Green tea group	Placebo group
	(n=30)	(n=24)
Age (years)	72.4 ± 4.2	72.6 ± 5.2
BMI (kg/m^2)	23.9 ± 3.1	22.5 ± 4.4
Body fat (%)	31.5 ± 7.9	32.8 ± 5.7
Skeletal muscle (kg)	18.4 ± 4.2	18.1 ± 2.5
Basal Metabolism (kcal/d)	1120.4 ± 84.2	1122.1 ± 80.9

Abbreviation: BMI, Body mass index.

Age, BMI, body fat, skeletal muscle and basal metabolism were not significantly different between the two groups; they were not overweight. Among the subjects analyzed, 4 women (16.7%) in the green tea group and 3 women (12.5%) in the placebo group were diagnosed with an osteoporosis defined T-score (<-2.5). Also, 24 women (80.0%) in the green tea group and 21 women (87.5%) in the placebo group were diagnosed with low bone mass level (T-score between -1.0 and -2.5). Figure 1 shows that a 5 month dietary intake of vitamin D (placebo group) increased bone mass ($p<0.05$), and dietary intake of GTE and vitamin D greatly increased bone mass ($p<0.01$). The number of women diagnosed as having a normal bone mass level (T-score > -1) increased from 0 to 2 in the placebo group and from 2 to 6 in the green tea group, and the number of women diagnosed with osteoporosis decreased from 4 to 1 in the green tea group. These results suggested that green tea and vitamin D may be beneficial in mitigating bone loss of this population.

Animal Studies

Ovariectomized female rats have been studied as a clinical animal model for postmenopausal osteoporosis. OVX rats showed significantly decreased bone strength compared with SHAM rats (Fig. 2). Supplementation of EGCG suppressed the bone loss induced in the OVX rats (Fig. 2). In the results obtained from the three-point bending test of the femur, EGCG caused a greater increase in the amount of pressure required to fracture the femur compared with OVX rats.

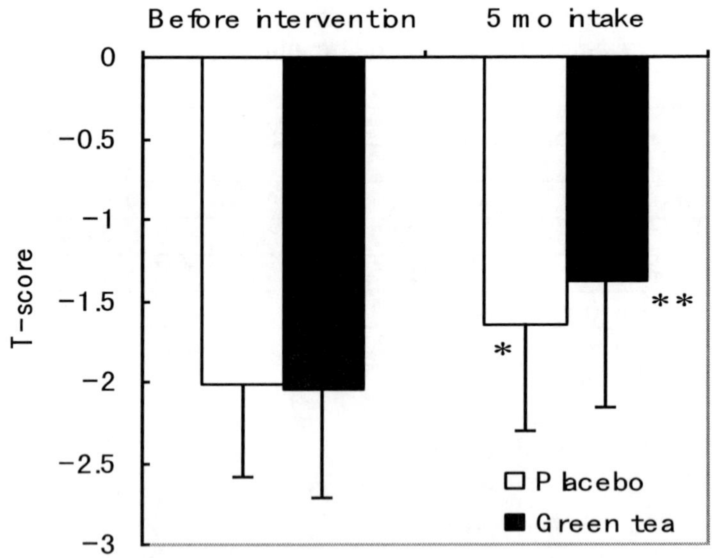

Figure 1. Effects of green tea extract and vitamin D on bone mineral density in elderly women. Results are presented as the mean ± SD: *, p<0.05, **, p<0.01 as compared with measurements before intervention.

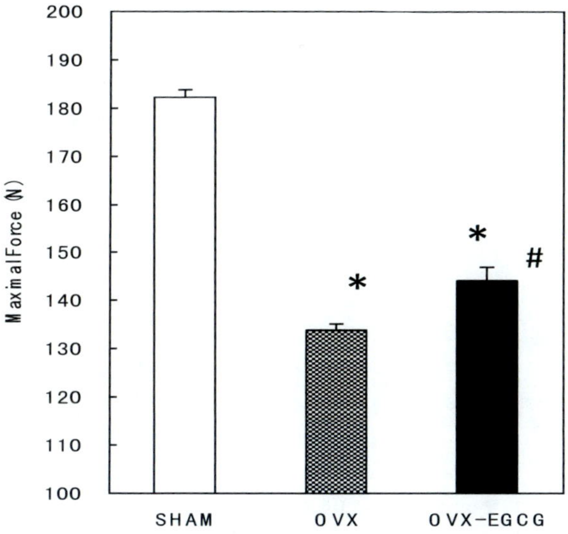

Figure 2. Effects of EGCG on femur bone strength in OVX rats. OVX rats were housed for 3 months and subjected to three-point bending tests. Results are presented as mean ± SEM of six experiments: **, p<0.01 as compared with SHAM, #, p<0.05 as compared between OVX and OVX-EGCG.

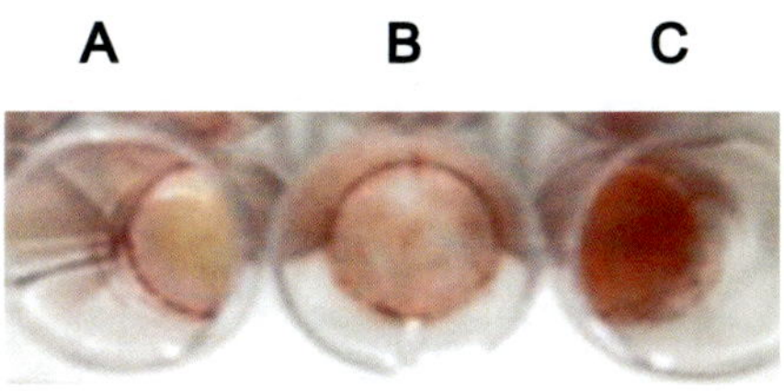

Figure 3. Effect of EGCG on mineralization of MC3T3-E1 cells. MC3T3-E1 cells were differentiated for 28 d. Level of mineralization was evaluated by alizarin red S staining in control group (A), differentiated group (B) and EGCG-treated differentiated group (C).

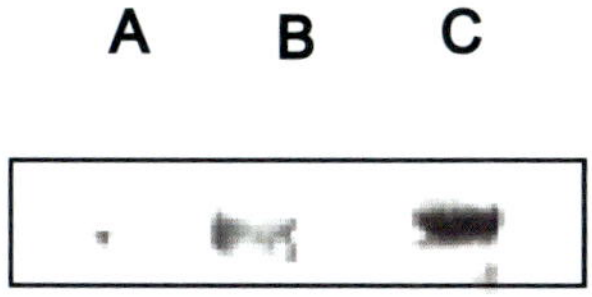

Figure 4. Effect of EGCG on expression of ERβ in MC3T3-E1 cells. MC3T3-E1 cells were differentiated for 28 d. Level of expression of ERβ was evaluated by Western blot analysis in control group (A), differentiated group (B) and EGCG-treated differentiated group (C).

Cellular Studies

Figure 3 shows the level of mineralization of MC3T3-E1 cells. The area stained red indicates the sites where calcium was deposited. The cells in the control group showed no mineralization nodule (A), but the cells in the presence of β-glycerophosphate and L-ascorbic acid formed nodules (B). EGCG activated and promoted mineralization of MC3T3-E1 cells (C), and suggested that EGCG helps to maintain bone mineral density. MC3T3-E1 cells have been reported to have ERβ for the differentiation of osteoblasts. Figure 4 shows the level of ERβ expression in MC3T3-E1 cells. Cells in the control group showed no expression of ERβ (A), but cells in the presence of β-glycerophosphate and L-ascorbic acid expressed ERβ (B). EGCG activated the expression of ERβ (C). These results suggest that EGCG stimulates osteoblastic differentiation via the expression of ERβ. There are many reports concerning the activated effect of natural products concluding that polyphenols are active in mineralization of MC3T3-E1 cells [12-14]. These results suggest that GTE containing polyphenol may be able to enhance bone formation.

Conclusion

We demonstrated in the present study that green tea ingestion may be beneficial in mitigating bone loss and decreasing osteoporotic fractural risk.

References

[1] National Institutes of Health. Osteoporosis Prevention, Diagnosis, and Therapy [online]. 2000 [cited 2000 March 27-29]. Available from: URL: http://consensus.nih.gov/2000/2000Osteoporosis111html.htm

[2] Orimo, H., Nakamura, T., & Fukunaga, M. (2006). *Japanese guidelines for the prevention and treatment of osteoporosis, Translated Abridged Edition*. Tokyo: Life Science Publishing.

[3] Kaptoge, S., Welch, A., McTaggart, A., Mulligan, A., Dalzell, N., Day, N. E., Bingham, S., Khaw, K. T., & Reeve, J. (2003). Effects of dietary nutrients and food groups on bone loss from the proximal femur in men

and women in the 7th and 8th decades of age. *Osteoporos Int.*, *14*, 418-428.

[4] Hardcastle, A. C., Aucott, L., Reid, D. M., & Macdonald, H. M. (2011). Associations between dietary flavonoid intakes and bone health in a Scottish population. *J Bone Miner Res.*, *26*, 941-947.

[5] Yang, C. S., & Landau, J. M. (2000). Effects of tea consumption on nutrition and health. *J Nutr.*, *130*, 2409-2412.

[6] Shen, C. L., Cao, J. J., Dagda, R. Y., Tenner, T. E. Jr, Chyu, M. C., & Yeh, J. K. (2011). Supplementation with green tea polyphenols improves bone microstructure and quality in aged, orchidectomized rats. *Calcif Tissue Int.*, *88*, 455-463.

[7] Shen, C. L., Wang, P., Guerrieri, J., Yeh, J. K., & Wang, J. S. (2008). Protective effect of green tea pollyphenols on bone loss in middle-aged female rats. *Osteoporos Int.*, *19*, 979-990.

[8] Shen, C. L., Yeh, J. K., Cao, J. J., Chyu, M. C., & Wang, J. S. (2011). Green tea and bone health: Evidence from laboratory studies. *Pharmacol Res.*, *64.*, 155-161.

[9] Hoover, P. A., Webber, C. E., Beaumont, L. F., & Blake, J. M. (1996). Postmenopausal bone mineral density: relationship to calcium intake, calcium absorption, residual estrogen, body composition, and physical activity. *Can J Physiol Pharmacol.*, *74*, 911-917.

[10] Muraki, S., Yamamoto, S., Ishibashi, H., Oka, H., Yoshimura, N., kawaguchi, H., & Nakamura, K. (2007). Diet and lifestyle associated with increased bone mineral density: cross-sectional study of Japanese elderly women at an osteoporosis outpatient clinic. *J Orthop Sci.*, *12*, 317-320.

[11] Mei, L., Mochizuki, M., & Hasegawa, N. (2012). Protective effect of Pycnogenol-R on ovariectomy-induced bone loss in rats. *Phytother Res.*, *26*, 153-155

[12] Ge, Y., Chen, D., Xie, L., & Zhang R. (2006). Enhancing effect of Daidzein on the differentiation and mineralization in mouse osteoblast-like MC3T3-E1 cells. *Yakugaku Zasshi*, *126*, 651-656.

[13] Lee, KH., & Choi. EM. (2005). Biochanin A stimulates osteoblastic differentiation and inhibits hydrogen peroxide-induced production of inflammatory mediators in MC3T3-E1 cell. *Biol Pharm Bull.*, *28*, 1948-1953.

[14] Ono,Y., Fukaya, Y., Imai, S., & Yamakuni, T. (2008). Benefical effects of Ajuga decumbens on osteoporosis and arthritis. *Biol Pharm Bull.*, *31*, 1199-1204.

In: Bone Loss
Editor: Kuo-Cheng Lu
ISBN: 978-1-62417-169-7

Chapter 8

HIP FRACTURES IN THE ELDERLY: A RECONSIDERATION

Juan D. Pedrera-Zamorano, Julián F. Calderón-García, Raúl Roncero-Martín, María del Carmen Costa-Fernández, José M. Morán and Jesús M. Lavado-García
Metabolic Bone Diseases Research Group. University of Extremadura.
Escuela de Enfermería y TO. Caceres, Spain

ABSTRACT

Hip fractures in the elderly are common and considered one of the most fatal fractures, resulting in impaired function, and are associated with a high rate of morbidity and mortality. The situation will clearly become worse because the continuous increase in life expectancy will cause a 3-fold rise in fracture incidence worldwide over the next 60 years, affecting women in particular. Hip fractures account for a large proportion ofdisability, death and medical costs associated with fall. Althougth age-related bone loss can be regarded as the main determinant in the risk of hip fracture in the elderly, not all hip fractures in elderly subjects are caused by osteoporosis, a concept that has not been given sufficient attention and is all too often overlooked. Because fracture treatment is expensive and rehabilitation is not always successful, effective prophylaxis offers the only hope of alleviating the enormous social burden of hip fractures. Preventive measures are the best and the most cost-effective means to minimize hip fractures.

BACKGROUND

Hip fracture is a common, morbid and costly health problem. It can cause substantial disability and even death. For a 50-year old Caucasian woman today, the risk of incurring a hip fracture over her remaining lifetime is approximately 17%. [1] The situation will clearly become worse because the continuous increase in life expectancy will cause a 3-fold rise in fracture incidence worldwide over the next 60 years, affecting women in particular. Multiple causes have been identified in hip fractures in the elderly (Figure 1), but the relative importance of social and anthropometric variables, vitamin D deficiency with secondary hyperparathyroidism, nutritional deficiency, and low bone mineral density (BMD), among other risk factors for hip fracture, has yet to be established. [2]

Age-related bone loss can be regarded as the main determinant in the risk of hip fracture in the elderly. However, not all hip fractures in elderly subjects are caused by osteoporosis. [3] Vitamin D deficiency may a key role in senile osteoporosis [4], as Jenkins et al. demonstrated 38 years ago. [5] This concept, however, has not been given sufficient attention and is all too often overlooked. This neglect has given rise to the generalized and erroneous assumption that all hip fractures in the elderly are due to osteoporosis, when in fact many, if not the majority, are caused by osteomalacia. In fact, some clinicians doubt that a fracture of the hip, femoral neck or intertrochanteric fractures, which are considered purely osteoporotic, share a common cause. [6]

OSTEOMALACIC *VERSUS* OSTEOPOROTIC HIP FRACTURE

Because fracture treatment is expensive and rehabilitation is not always successful, effective prophylaxis offers the only hope of alleviating the enormous social burden of hip fractures. Preventive measures are the best and the most cost-effective means to minimize hip fractures. Because hip fractures account for the greatest socioeconomic impact attributed to osteoporosis and because there is growing evidence that treatments can favorably impact hip fracture risk, it has been suggested that greater attention be paid to the management of hip fractures in the elderly. For this management to be effective, it is necessary to elucidate the causes of hip fracture. Apart from osteoporosis (i.e., loss of bone mass in the strict sense, with normal organic and mineral structure in the remaining bone), there is another though often forgotten cause of hip fracture, namely, osteomalacia. It is important not to overlook this cause of fracture because the incidence of osteomalacia can be reduced with suitable treatment, as has been demonstrated. [7] Daily supplementation with 400-800 IU vitamin D slightly decreases PTH secretion and increases bone mineral density at the femoral neck in elderly women. [8] Classifying hip fractures as either osteoporotic or osteomalacic, therefore, bears important implications, not only from the perspective of prevention through adequate forms of therapy but also from an epidemiological perspective. In a group of 570 healthy women (mean age 82.3+8.8(SD) years), 77.8% of patients with cervical and the 82.1% with trochanteric hip fracture showed serum 25(OH)D levels below 50 mmol/L. The serum 25(OH)D levels in these elderly women were associated with secondary hyperparathyroidism, and they increased bone turnover. [9] This situation can obviously induce an osteomalacic hip fracture, indicating that the prevalence of this type of fracture (approximately 77%) may be higher than that of fractures generally considered to be osteoporotic.

At other times, hip fractures in the elderly occur in normal bone mass and, therefore, in the absence of either osteoporosis or osteomalacia. In these instances, the cause is often attributed to a fall or, if independent of the intensity of a fall's impact, to geometric changes in the proximal femur (the angle of the femoral neck with respect to its diaphysis and/or to the greater length of the femur neck itself). Other variables dependent on the individual may also be identified as the cause, such as height (the taller the subject, the longer the femoral neck and the greater the impact upon falling and vice versa) or body index (the lower the body mass index, the lower the cushioning effect on impact and vice versa) and the ability of the subject to protect her/himself from the fall as a function of the general state of help of the individual (e.g., hemiplegia) or whether the individual is on medication that might enhance or minimize his/her capacity to react (e.g., ansiolitic axiolytic drugs). [10] Approximately 30% of people aged over 65 years living in the community fall at least once a year, with an even higher rate in nursing homes. Many of these falls lead to fractures, the most serious of which are hip fractures. [11] Falls, therefore, constitute an important factor that can lead to hip fracture in normal bone mass, or with osteoporosis and/or osteomalacia. Together with the fall, as we have said above, the other important factors to be taken into account as determinants of hip fracture are the individual's height, the length of the femoral neck and the individual's body constitution, or BMI. [12]

In turn, hip fractures in the elderly that are secondary to osteoporosis may occur if the osteoporosis develops because of dietary deficiencies of a general nature or related to specific nutrients. This topic, however, is subject to ongoing debate. [13;14] Nutritional deficiencies, in a broad sense, may be important, and as we have pointed out earlier, this topic has been extensively dealt with in the literature. [15;16] It has been proposed that BMD significantly correlates with serum albumin. [17] Thus, poor nutritional status evident in inadequate dietary intake, reduced serum albumin and decreased body mass and soft tissues, thus increasing the risk of subsequent hip fracture. Moreover, recently it has been proposed that serum albumin level by bromocresol green assay could overestimate the serum albumin level, and hence underestimate the percentage of subjects with protein energy malnutrition in hip fractured patients. [18]

Other factures may be related to lifestyle and habit, as evidenced by different hip fracture rates observed in different races and geographical locations. These factors have been highlighted in studies in the United States that have examined Asian and Latin American populations. [19-21] Age-adjusted hip fracture incidence was lower for Chinese, Japanese and Korean Asian American groups compared with Caucasians. [22;23] Studies conducted in Europe bear out the same hypothesis. In Europe, there is a marked geographical distribution in the incidence of hip fractures. Indeed, the differences in incidences between communities are greater than the differences in incidences between the sexes within the same community. This geographical effect suggests that the importance of gonadal insufficiency in women has been overemphasized and that other factors, most likely related to genetic or lifestyle factors affecting peak bone density, account for the differences in the incidence of hip fracture detected from one community to another.

CONCLUSION

Some hip fractures occur in diminished bone mass in the presence of primary or secondary osteoporosis and/or osteomalacia. In these cases, the subject breaks a hip and falls. Other fractures, however, occur in normal bone mass when the subject falls and then breaks a hip. As we know, the number of hip fracture incidents is increasing daily, generating serious health problems throughout the world. [1;24] As we have stated above, there are multiple causes of hip fractures in the elderly, and it would be of great interest to have an epidemiological breakdown of each of these causes. While difficult, this task is not impossible. Compiling these statistics would mean that those of us who are interested in the topic would have to define the etiology of the hip fractures that we see to avoid the mistake of diagnosing hip fractures almost unanimously as osteoporotic.

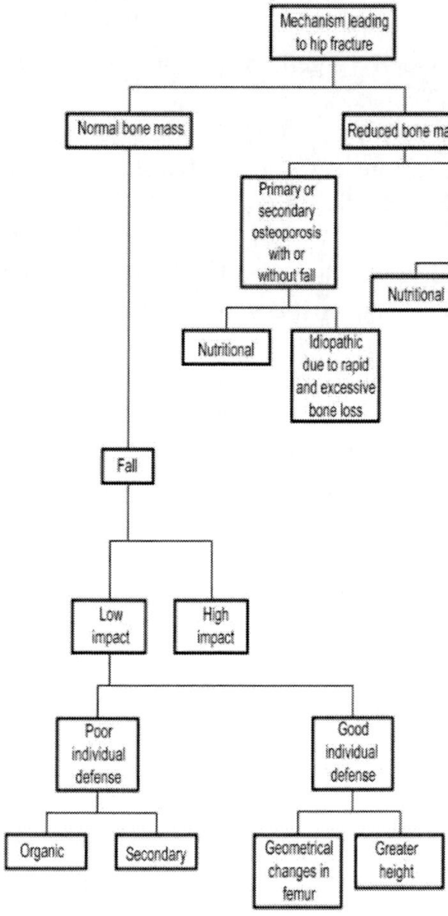

Figure 1. Multiple causes of hip fractures in the elderly.

References

[1] Johnell O, Kanis J. Epidemiology of osteoporotic fractures. *Osteoporos Int* 2005 Mar;16 Suppl 2:S3-S7.

[2] Kristensen M. Factors affecting functional prognosis of patients with hip fracture. *Eur J Phys Rehabil Med* 2011 Jun;47(2):257-64.

[3] Tanner DA, Kloseck M, Crilly RG, Chesworth B, Gilliland J. Hip fracture types in men and women change differently with age. *BMC Geriatr* 2010;10:12.

[4] Boonen S, Dejaeger E, Vanderschueren D, Venken K, Bogaerts A, Verschueren S, et al. Osteoporosis and osteoporotic fracture occurrence and prevention in the elderly: a geriatric perspective. *Best Pract Res Clin Endocrinol Metab* 2008 Oct;22(5):765-85.

[5] Jenkins DH, Roberts JG, Webster D, Williams EO. Osteomalacia in elderly patients with fracture of the femoral neck. A clinico-pathological study. *J Bone Joint Surg Br* 1973 Aug;55(3):575-80.

[6] Cornwall R, Gilbert MS, Koval KJ, Strauss E, Siu AL. Functional outcomes and mortality vary among different types of hip fractures: a function of patient characteristics. *Clin Orthop Relat Res* 2004 Aug;(425):64-71.

[7] Sawka AM, Ismaila N, Cranney A, Thabane L, Kastner M, Gafni A, et al. A scoping review of strategies for the prevention of hip fracture in elderly nursing home residents. *PLoS One* 2010;5(3):e9515.

[8] Karkkainen M, Tuppurainen M, Salovaara K, Sandini L, Rikkonen T, Sirola J, et al. Effect of calcium and vitamin D supplementation on bone mineral density in women aged 65-71 years: a 3-year randomized population-based trial (OSTPRE-FPS). *Osteoporos Int* 2010 Dec;21(12):2047-55.

[9] Fisher A, Srikusalanukul W, Davis M, Smith P. Hip fracture type: important role of parathyroid hormone (PTH) response to hypovitaminosis D. *Bone* 2010 Aug;47(2):400-7.

[10] Benetos IS, Babis GC, Zoubos AB, Benetou V, Soucacos PN. Factors affecting the risk of hip fractures. *Injury* 2007 Jul;38(7):735-44.

[11] Blain H, Blain A, Trechot P, Jeandel C. [The role of drugs in falls in the elderly. Epidemiologic aspects]. *Presse Med* 2000 Apr 1;29(12):673-80.

[12] Pillai A, Eranki V, Shenoy R, Hadidi M. Age Related Incidence and Early Outcomes of Hip Fractures: A Prospective Cohort Study of 1177 patients. *J Orthop Surg Res* 2011;6(1):5.

[13] Benetou V, Orfanos P, Zylis D, Sieri S, Contiero P, Tumino R, et al. Diet and hip fractures among elderly Europeans in the EPIC cohort. *Eur J Clin Nutr* 2011 Jan;65(1):132-9.

[14] Misra D, Berry SD, Broe KE, McLean RR, Cupples LA, Tucker KL, et al. Does dietary protein reduce hip fracture risk in elders? The Framingham Osteoporosis Study. *Osteoporos Int* 2011 Jan;22(1):345-9.

[15] Mak JC, Cameron ID, March LM. Evidence-based guidelines for the management of hip fractures in older persons: an update. *Med J Aust* 2010 Jan 4;192(1):37-41.

[16] Pedrera JD, Canal ML, Postigo S, Lavado J, Hernandez ER, Rico H. Phalangeal bone ultrasound and its possible correlation with nutrient in an area of high protein intake. *Ann Nutr Metab* 2001;45(2):86-90.

[17] Miyanishi K, Jingushi S, Torisu T. Mortality after hip fracture in Japan: the role of nutritional status. *J Orthop Surg* (Hong Kong) 2010 Dec;18(3):265-70.

[18] Nakano T, Kuwabara A, Tanaka K. Overestimated serum albumin levels in patients with hip fracture. *Clin Nutr* 2011 Apr;30(2):261.

[19] Wu Q, Lefante JJ, Rice JC, Magnus JH. Age, race, weight, and gender impact normative values of bone mineral density. *Gend Med* 2011 Jun;8(3):189-201.

[20] Cauley JA. Defining ethnic and racial differences in osteoporosis and fragility fractures. *Clin Orthop Relat Res* 2011 Jul;469(7):1891-9.

[21] Megyesi MS, Hunt LM, Brody H. A critical review of racial/ethnic variables in osteoporosis and bone density research. *Osteoporos Int* 2011 Jun;22(6):1669-79.

[22] Fang J, Freeman R, Jeganathan R, Alderman MH. Variations in hip fracture hospitalization rates among different race/ethnicity groups in New York City. *Ethn Dis* 2004;14(2):280-4.

[23] Lauderdale DS, Rathouz PJ. Body mass index in a US national sample of Asian Americans: effects of nativity, years since immigration and socioeconomic status. *Int J Obes Relat Metab Disord* 2000 Sep;24(9):1188-94.

[24] Pedrera Zamorano JD, Bote Mohedano JL, Lavado Garcia JM, Rodriguez Dominguez MT, Hernandez Diaz ER, Rico LH. [Incidence and prevalence of hip fractures in the province of Caceres and their evolutionary trend]. *Rev Clin Esp* 2004 Sep;204(9):448-51.

INDEX

C

D

E

F

G

H

I

K

L

M

N

O

P

R

S

T

V

W

Z